# THE PHILOSOPHY
# AND PSYCHOLOGY
# OF SENSATION

* *

By CHARLES HARTSHORNE
*Assistant Professor of Philosophy, the University of Chicago*

* *

WIPF & STOCK · Eugene, Oregon

Wipf and Stock Publishers
199 W 8th Ave, Suite 3
Eugene, OR 97401

The Philosophy and Psychology of Sensation
By Hartshorne, Charles H.
ISBN 13: 978-1-62564-579-1
Publication date 1/10/2014
Previously published by University of Chicago Press, 1934

*All that life offers any man from which to start his thinking or his striving is a fact. And if this universe is one universe, if it is so far thinkable that you can pass in reason from one part of it to another, it does not matter very much what that fact is. . . . . Your business as thinkers is to make plainer the way from something to the whole of things; to show the rational connection between your fact and the frame of the universe.*

CHIEF JUSTICE OLIVER WENDELL HOLMES

**

*The essence of the sensory intuitive lies not in what separates the senses but in what unites them—with each other, with all even the non-sensory aspects of our experience, and with everything without us which is there to be experienced.*

ERICH M. VON HORNBOSTEL

**

*Of the continuity of intrinsic qualities of feeling we can now form but a feeble conception. The development of the human mind has practically extinguished all feelings, except a few sporadic kinds, sounds, colors, smells, warmth, etc., which now appear to be disconnected and disparate. In the case of colors, there is a tri-dimensional spread of feelings. Originally, all feelings may have been connected in the same way. . . . .*

CHARLES S. PEIRCE

**

*The question of the proper description of the species of qualities termed "sensa" is important. Unfortunately the learned tradition of philosophy has missed their main characteristic, which is their enormous emotional significance. The vicious notion has been introduced of mere receptive entertainment, which for no obvious reason by reflection acquires an affective tone. The very opposite is the true explanation. The true doctrine of sense-perceptions is that the qualitative characters of affective tones inherent in the bodily functionings are transmuted into the characters of regions. . . . . This is the reason of the definite aesthetic attitude imposed by sense-perception.*

A. N. WHITEHEAD

**

*Color is a spirit upon things by which they become intelligible to the spirit.*

WALTER PATER

**

*For a scientific man a philosophy is not a creed but a program.*

J. B. S. HALDANE

# PREFACE

THIS book presents a theory of the sensory qualities. The theory may be called, for brevity's sake, the doctrine of the "affective continuum." It was first conceived as an attempt to solve certain problems of a philosophical character. But it was natural that the treatment which the subject of sensation has received in experimental psychology should have come to occupy an ever larger place in the inquiry. In the end it is the topic of sensation as a whole and however approached with which I have sought to deal. Being a philosopher by training, I have not scrupled to give serious consideration to speculations which to a psychologist might seem of negligible value (e.g., in chaps. iii and vi); but, on the other hand, I have assembled a considerable quantity of experimental data (chaps. ii, iv, vii) which hitherto has lain scattered through the psychological literature, largely unknown to philosophers, and apparently not as yet correlated and seen as a whole even by psychologists. In short, I have sought evidence and suggestions bearing upon the question "What is sensation?" wherever such evidence or suggestions could conceivably be found.

It will be obvious that I have been much influenced by two philosopher-scientists who appear to have a good deal in common—Charles S. Peirce and Professor A. N. Whitehead. In a general way I take my conclusions to be, for the most part, compatible with their views. The central idea of this book occurred to me, however, at a time when I was quite ignorant of these philosophies. An earlier obligation was to the philosophical idealists, especially Royce, Creighton, and my former teacher, Professor William Ernest Hocking. If, indeed, "idealism" means that reality is essentially spiritual, and if "spiritual" means, as I think it should, irreducibly socio-emotional, or having to do with "love," then the most general conclusion which I feel warranted in drawing from the evidence supporting the affective continuum is an idealistic one. But many of the chief historical suggestions of the word "idealism" I should as little wish to defend as the "realists."

The psychological sources upon which I have principally drawn are not confined to any particular school or group, but I feel especially indebted to the late L. T. Troland, to Professor E. G. Boring, and to Julius Pikler. Only in the third case, however, does this indebtedness involve any close similarity of psychological outlook.

With the current behavioristic emphasis in psychology (of which a recent expression is Boring's *Physical Dimensions of Consciousness*) I have sufficient sympathy to believe that unless conceptions of sensation can, sooner or later, be made physiologically definite, they are probably of little value. Yet it has seemed to me that the failure so far to verify conclusively a single major hypothesis—with one exception which, as we shall see presently, only reinforces the rule—concerning the operation of the several sense organs may derive in part from an erroneous analysis of the primary data of the problem, the sense qualities as immediately given.

My attempt has been to show that erroneous modes of sensory analysis have indeed prevailed, but that other modes are beginning to appear (Pikler, and Marston, Daly, and Marston) of which the concept of the affective continuum is a partly new version. From this concept a number of physiological consequences follow whose experimental testing is probably only a matter of time. For instance, the recent experiments (beginning with those by Wever and Bray) upon the relation of pitch to frequency of nervous conduction are deducible from the analysis of auditory quality which I had previously worked out, while they certainly are not deducible, except in an indirect and uncertain fashion, from traditional introspective analyses.

The first five chapters are predominantly argumentative. Chapters i and ii furnish, it is hoped, a sufficient refutation of the supposed axiom that sensory qualities are necessarily inexplicable, for they show that a theory to explain them is quite conceivable. Chapter ii attacks the prevalent alternative to this theory as inconsistent with the facts and as belonging to a pattern of theory elsewhere discredited in science. In chapter iii it is argued that the conflict of philosophical opinions concerning the nature of the physical world cannot be settled unless a new approach to the problem of sense data can be found, and that with such an approach a reasonable measure of agreement might be attained. Chapter iv depicts psychology as standing at the threshold of a new generalization concerning the nature of sensory experience, and indeed concerning mind generally. Chapter v is an attempt to derive the affective continuum from the data of aesthetics, and to show its value for this study.

The last three chapters are largely expository, and are to be regarded as highly tentative. Chapter vi might be called a deduction of the dimensions of quality. The problem of the nature of mind is reduced to a conception of variables of "feeling of feeling," social feeling as such, and their possible values. Sensation is exhibited as but a certain portion of the range of these values. In chapter vii these conceptions are applied to the details of sensory experience. Chapter viii indicates some of the consequences for biology and cosmology.

I am indebted to Professor Edwin Arthur Burtt, of Cornell University; Professor Everett W. Hall, of Leland Stanford University; and Professors Arthur C. Bills and Ralph W. Gerard, of the University of Chicago, for helpful suggestions; to my wife, Dorothy C. Hartshorne, for the host of improvements in style and organization which are due to her skilful editorial assistance; and, finally, to all my former teachers in philosophy and psychology at Harvard. For the index, as well as for friendly encouragement and criticism, my grateful thanks are due to Professor Clyde B. Cooper.

My object in publishing this book is in part to acquire a new indebtedness—to those who may be moved to join with me in an inquiry the present outcome of which is only less baffling to me than it is likely to be to the average reader. I cannot see my way back to the prevailing ideas of sensation—these ideas seem visibly waning in influence and full of absurdity—but neither can I escape the feeling that some portion or other of the alternative I have set up is likewise unsatisfactory. How large is that portion, and what can be done to reduce it? Or is science not yet in a position to deal with the problem? That my own method is insufficiently scientific, objective, I am aware. Yet if it serves to induce those capable of bettering it to do so, it will not have failed in its purpose.

CHARLES HARTSHORNE

UNIVERSITY OF CHICAGO
February, 1934

## ACKNOWLEDGMENTS

For permission to reprint the quotation on page v from *Adventures of Ideas* by A. N. Whitehead, grateful acknowledgment is made to the publishers, The Macmillan Company; for the quotation on page v from *Speeches* by Oliver Wendell Holmes, to Little, Brown and Company; for the quotations on pages v and 209 from *Chance, Love and Logic* by Charles S. Peirce, and the quotation on page 107 from *The Nature of Intelligence* by L. L. Thurstone, to Harcourt Brace and Company; for the quotation on page 243 from *The Causes of Evolution* by J. B. S. Haldane, to Harper and Brothers; and for the quotation on page 190 from *Collected Papers of Charles Sanders Peirce*, Volume II (ed. Hartshorne and Weiss), and the quotation on page 243, *ibid.*, Volume I, to the Department of Philosophy of Harvard University.

# CONTENTS

| CHAPTER | PAGE |
|---|---|
| I. Two Theories of Sensation | 1 |
|    Section 1. Sensation: A Concept in Flux | 1 |
|    Section 2. Definition of the Affective Continuum | 5 |
|    Section 3. The Passing of Materialism | 10 |
|    Section 4. Qualities and the New Doctrine of Analysis | 20 |
| II. An Unscientific Hypothesis | 29 |
|    Section 5. The Logical Structure of the Current Theory | 29 |
|       A. The Criterion of Simplicity | 29 |
|       B. Knowing, Feeling, and Willing | 36 |
|       C. The Geometry of Color | 40 |
|    Section 6. The Facts | 49 |
|       A. Pain, Temperature, and Affection | 49 |
|       B. Pitch and Brightness | 59 |
|       C. Further Intersense Analogies | 74 |
|       D. Modes and Fusion | 76 |
|       E. Synesthesia | 77 |
|    Section 7. The Failure to Produce Agreement | 85 |
| III. The Deadlock in Contemporary Philosophy | 87 |
|    Section 8. The Appeal to the Sense Datum | 87 |
|    Section 9. The Status of Tertiary Qualities | 95 |
|    Section 10. Quality and Interest | 99 |
|    Section 11. The Philosopher as Observer | 102 |
| IV. The Conflict of Opinions in Psychology | 107 |
|    Section 12. Sensation and Feeling | 107 |
|    Section 13. Objective Feelings | 117 |
|    Section 14. Is Feeling an Attribute of Sensation? | 124 |
|    Section 15. Subjective Feelings | 126 |
|    Section 16. Alleged Criteria of the Distinctness of Sensation and Feeling | 130 |
|    Section 17. How Feelings Become Sensations | 135 |
|    Section 18. The Persistence of Associational and Faculty Psychologies | 136 |
|    Section 19. Atomism in Psychology | 138 |
|    Section 20. Dimensional Theories of Sensation | 146 |
|    Section 21. Behavior, Gestalt, and Affective Continuity | 152 |

## CONTENTS

| CHAPTER | PAGE |
|---|---|

**V. DUALISM IN AESTHETICS** . . . . . . . . . . . . . 159
    Section 22. The Premises of Aesthetics . . . . . . . 159
    Section 23. Expression and Association . . . . . . 169
    Section 24. Expression and Immanence . . . . . . 175
    Section 25. Quality and Pattern . . . . . . . . 182

**VI. THE DIMENSIONS OF EXPERIENCE** . . . . . . . . . 190
    Section 26. Dimensional Analysis in Science . . . . . 190
    Section 27. The Social Continuum . . . . . . . . 191
    Section 28. The Ultimate Dimensions . . . . . . . 194
    Section 29. Space: The Primary Qualities . . . . . 196
    Section 30. The Affective Continuum . . . . . . . 200
    Section 31. Vagueness: The Evolution of Qualities . . . 207

**VII. THE DIMENSIONS OF SENSATION** . . . . . . . . . 209
    Section 32. Color . . . . . . . . . . . . . 209
    Section 33. Sound . . . . . . . . . . . . . 225
    Section 34. Touch, Temperature, and Pain . . . . . 234
    Section 35. Taste and Smell . . . . . . . . . . 236
    Section 36. The General Question . . . . . . . . 241

**VIII. SENSATION AND ENVIRONMENT** . . . . . . . . . 243
    Section 37. The Psycho-physical Problem . . . . . . 243
    Section 38. Sense Qualities and Adaptation . . . . . 250
            A. Vision and Behavior . . . . . . . . 253
            B. Hearing . . . . . . . . . . . . 257
            C. Thermal Sensations . . . . . . . . 259
            D. The Chemical Senses and Pleasure and Pain . 261
    Section 39. The Verification of Panpsychism . . . . . 263
    Section 40. Conclusion: Some Predictions . . . . . 266

**APPENDIX**

A. THE AFFECTIVE CONTINUUM IN THEOLOGY . . . . . . 271

B. WHY THE CURRENT DOCTRINE OF PITCH AND LOUDNESS AROSE . 273

C. BRIGHTNESS AS A UNIVERSAL ATTRIBUTE . . . . . . . 277

D. GOETHE'S *Farbenlehre* . . . . . . . . . . . . 278

E. BIBLIOGRAPHICAL NOTE . . . . . . . . . . . . 280

INDEX . . . . . . . . . . . . . . . . . . 283

# CHAPTER I

# TWO THEORIES OF SENSATION

**\*\***

*Science is a struggle with what is as yet unintelligible, and this struggle is its very life.*

J. S. Haldane

*Logical analysis is not dissection but relation.*

C. I. Lewis

**\*\***

### SECTION I. SENSATION: A CONCEPT IN FLUX

THE present age is frequently characterized as one of intellectual change striking at the roots of things. Among the concepts which are cited as subjects of such change is that of "sensation." The old notion of sensory "elements" of mind, elaborated by Locke, Hume, and the earlier psychologists, is now regarded as obsolete, one of the many oversimplifications which we owe to seventeenth- and eighteenth-century rationalism.

There is a striking fact about this widespread opinion, however; namely, that, as usually expressed, it is largely negative in character. We are told often enough what sensation is no longer thought to be; we are told far less about what, according to the newer concept on its positive side, a sensation after all is. For instance, we are told that a sensation, like all the factors in consciousness, is not to be regarded in complete abstraction from the remaining factors—emotions, ideas, memories, motor responses, and the rest. But of just how this supposedly more integral view really affects our understanding of sensory experiences we are not, for the most part, given any but the most fragmentary indications.[1]

---

[1] Two interesting and important exceptions to this statement are found in *Integrative Psychology* (1931), by W. M. Marston, C. D. King, and E. H. Marston; and in the writings of Julius Pikler of Budapest (*Schriften zur Anpassungstheorie des Empfindungsvorganges* [1919-26]). See below, sec. 20.

How different are the changes which the physicists have effected! They are not content with telling us that space must not be considered except in relation to time; they tell us just how, in practice, time measurements enter into and affect space measurements. Now analogous developments in regard to the new concept of sensation are not wholly wanting; but there are reasons for thinking that psychologists are at the beginning of these changes, in comparison with the physicists, who, let us say, are well in the middle of theirs. The philosophy and psychology of sensation, in short, have fallen somewhat behind in the general march of ideas. But so, you may reply, have philosophy and psychology in general. Perhaps, indeed, the comparison with physics is unfair; perhaps it is due to the very nature of sensations, as "ineffable" or "simple" intuitions, that, even with the aid of the new conceptions, there is little positively to be said about them.

And yet, however possible or probable this may appear to be, are we not justified in reflecting upon the implications of such a supposition? If it is true that "all knowledge of the real world comes to us through the senses"—and we need not commit the "sensationalist fallacy" to recognize that at least all detailed and precise knowledge comes to us in this way—then, or in so far, must our conception of reality depend upon two things: on the one hand, upon those special features of the sensory report which are studied by the special sciences; and, on the other, upon whatever of its more general features, whatever characters of sensation as such, philosophy or psychology may bring to light. If we know in a general way how the world appears to us sensuously, we are then, but only then, in a position to consider the most general characters which can reasonably be ascribed to the world which appears. If there are no such clearly ascertainable general characters of sensation, then it seems there can be no positive conceptions of a general kind about the physical world. How, for instance, can we interpret the new concepts of physics according to which physical reality transcends sensuous representation, if we do not know what sensuous representation is? The rôle of the sensory factor in experience is too fundamental for us lightly to accept a conception which threatens to throw into eternal obscurity the innumerable problems in which this factor is involved. To take another such problem, how shall we clarify the age-old question of the "supersensible" objects of religion, if we do not know what "sensible" means?

The signs are indeed many that the whole system of knowledge is at present distorted and confused by the lack of adequate analysis of the sensory concept. Of course, it can hardly be supposed that so old and familiar an object of reflection, so accessible to the experience of everyone, should require for its analysis ideas which have hitherto occurred to no one. But is it not possible that, although the correct ideas are already current, they are rendered ineffective, partly by the weight of traditionally more accredited ideas, and partly by the circumstance that those who entertain the needed conceptions fall, as a natural result of modern specialization, into two classes: those who are interested in special cases and problems of detail, and have not as yet ventured to generalize broadly; and those whose interest is in ideas of the uttermost generality, but who have for the most part not concerned themselves with specific applications and verifications? In short, we have empirical psychologists, together with such philosophers as favor the piecemeal descriptive method, on the one hand, and metaphysicians, for whom even such a problem as sensation is only a corner of their domain, on the other. The history of science shows that it is the interplay of bold speculation with the meticulous exploration of facts which alone brings satisfying results. It is particularly at such a time of transition as the present that the two types of thought may come most fruitfully into contact.

It is significant that in regard to few subjects of inquiry has there been such a complete separation between the experimental and the speculative approaches. Philosophers would be ashamed of an ignorance of physics equal to that which they betray of recent findings of psychology in regard to sensory problems; which problems they nevertheless discuss no less frequently than those connected with physics. And although physicists pay but scant attention to philosophical views, they are not, I believe—and I am thinking of the known philosophical interests of such men as Einstein or Planck—quite so indifferent to them at the present time as are investigators of the psychology and physiology of sensory processes. Above all, it seems worth noting that the fundamental hypothesis of physics, the atomic theory, was originally a product of pure speculation indulged in many centuries before scientific verification was possible, so that, in so far as physics is our guide, we should at least be open to the possibility that the basic generalization which psychology, far more than physics, still lacks might be in part suggested by more or less ancient philosophical theories.

One aim of this book is to show that there does exist in philosophical literature a tradition which might indeed supply to psychology something like the aid which the atomic theory furnished to physics. This tradition is necessarily more subtle than Greek atomism, and for this and other reasons, including the tyranny of the successful doctrine of physical atomism over modern thought, has been relatively neglected.

In considering the possible value of philosophy for psychology, we should remember that there are philosophies and philosophies. The fear of metaphysics which now reigns in psychology must be interpreted in relation to the fact that the metaphysics which characterized the period in which experimental psychology arose has since been largely displaced in philosophy by a new type of thought, far more intimately inspired by the progress of natural science, and deserving, therefore, a very different respect. Indeed, the distrust and consequent neglect of metaphysics occasioned by the failure of eighteenth- and nineteenth-century world-views is one cause of the subconscious persistence of those very views. I believe we may say that if there is a certain set of metaphysical ideas whose prestige in the last century was owing to gaps in scientific knowledge which in the present century have been removed, then the two most promising places to look for the continued influence of these ideas is, on the one hand, among philosophers with a contempt for science, and, on the other, among psychologists—that is to say, practitioners of a science in which the demonstration of error against prejudice is peculiarly difficult—with a contempt for philosophy.

The conclusion is that a resolute attempt, such as this book professes to embody, to judge psychological and philosophical concepts of sensation in the light, so far as possible, of the totality of vital intellectual tendencies of the age, and of the ages, is by no means a superfluous undertaking. As the inquiry is arduous and complex, it may be serviceable to set down immediately the general goal toward which the argument moves, in the form of statements to be considered rather as hypotheses for later verification or correction than as doctrines to be accepted or rejected as they stand. A fundamental drift of ideas, such as contemporary thought discloses, cannot be safely evaluated in piecemeal fashion. It is only when the whole panorama is before one that the significance of particular features can be discerned.

### SECTION 2. DEFINITION OF THE AFFECTIVE CONTINUUM

The thesis of this book, negatively stated, is as follows: The currently accepted principles of scientific research and explanation, as well as the most characteristic ideas of contemporary philosophy, have not as yet been applied, with the thoroughness which the problem merits, to the question of the nature and distribution of the qualities immediately given in sensation, such as "red," "sour," or "warm"; and as a result the conceptions still generally held regarding these qualities conflict with the recognized criteria of a fruitful scientific hypothesis, or of an acceptable philosophical idea.

The comprehension of the greatest possible range of facts under the intelligible unity of the fewest and simplest general principles, such as is sought for everywhere in science, is achieved in the prevalent psychological and philosophical theories concerning sensation only in somewhat the same unsatisfactory way as it was in the Ptolemaic astronomy or in pre-evolutionary biology. The known facts, that is to say, are summed up in a cumbersome complexity of loosely interwoven ideas, from which further facts can seldom be deduced, and some of the deductions from which actually conflict with the facts already known.

The positive statement of the thesis to be considered may be formulated thus: the application of scientific and rational principles to the sensory qualities results in a new theory of these "immediate data of consciousness," considered both in themselves and in relation to their physical stimuli, organic conditions, biological significance, and evolutionary origin. This theory is characterized by the importance which it assigns to five fundamental conceptions:

1. Mathematical *continuity*
2. Aesthetic meaning or *affective tone*
3. The fundamentally *social* character of experience
4. Biological *adaptiveness*
5. *Evolution* from a common origin.

If each of these conceptions be embodied in an assertion indicating roughly its significance for the theory, we have the following five theses:

1. The type of relation existing between colors, whereby one is connected with or shades into another through intermediaries, can be generalized so as to connect qualities from different senses (e.g., a color and a sound) or from different elementary classes (e.g., secondary and tertiary qualities). This is contradictory to the almost universally accepted Helmholtzian dictum[2] that qualities from different sensory "modes" cannot be compared, but are irreducibly heterogeneous; further, it is the contradictory of the doctrine of the irreducible distinct-

[2] "Between sensory impressions of diverse kinds occur two distinct degrees of difference; first, a more fundamental one between impressions which belong to different senses, such as blue, sweet, warm, high-pitched; this difference I call one in the *modality* of the sensation. It is so profound that it excludes every transition from one to another, every relationship of greater or less resemblance. Whether, for example, sweet is more like blue or red, can simply not be asked. The second, less fundamental kind of difference, is that between sensations of the same sense .... [in regard to this difference] transition and comparison are possible" (Helmholtz, *Handbuch der physiologischen Optik* [2d ed., 1896], p. 584). The passage—which states with admirable precision, though without mention of any evidence, the doctrine I wish to call in question—is omitted but not corrected in later editions, including the English translation. The idea continues, however, to dominate the textbooks, still without critical discussion of the evidence upon which, one would suppose, it is believed to rest.

ness of sensory qualities and affective tones; and, finally, of the doctrine of an irreducible difference in kind between awareness and its contents.

It must, however, be noted that not all the intermediaries spoken of above are asserted to occur in actual experience. The essential point is that differences are matters of degree, whether or not all possible degrees can be found in the existent world.

2. The "affective" tonality, the aesthetic or tertiary quality, usually supposed to be merely "associated with" a given sensory quality is, in part at least, identical with that quality, one with its nature or essence. Thus, the "gaiety" of yellow (the peculiar highly specific gaiety) is the yellowness of the yellow. The two are identical in that the "yellowness" is the unanalyzed and but denotatively identified $x$ of which the "gaiety" is the essential description or analysis. (This description is extremely crude, vague, and partial—there is much more to be said concerning the yellowness of the yellow, and there is also this truth in the doctrine that such a quality is ineffable, namely, that a complete and perfect description of it is indeed beyond the power of language.)

Affective tone (Whitehead's "feeling-value") is thus the stuff of which the entire content of consciousness is composed. Although this tenet is in opposition to the prevalent associational view of aesthetic phenomena, it is shown to be compatible with the accredited facts of aesthetic association, and indeed to endow the association principle in some respects with an even greater explanatory power than that now conceded to it.[3]

The words "affective," "feeling," etc., require preliminary definition. If one limits, as it is probably best to do, the term "emotion" to feelings involving marked consciousness of intrabodily activities such as are emphasized in the James-Lange theory, then a color sensation is not emotional. It may, nevertheless, resemble emotion in certain respects; these respects I group under the name "feeling." "Affection"—pleasantness-unpleasantness—I regard as one among several of the respects in question, one among a number of dimensions of feeling. The

[3] See secs. 23, 38.

failure of previous multidimensional views of feeling, such as that of Wundt, I ascribe partly to the prevalence of a non-social conception of mind, partly to the dualistic conception of sensation and feeling, and partly to the conception of non-dimensional as well as dimensional qualitative differences—in other words, to the half-hearted way in which the idea of continuity has been applied in psychology.

3. Experience is social throughout, to its uttermost fragments or "elements." Its every mode is a mode of sociability. Thus, for example, the very objectivity or over-against-us character of sensations, particularly visual, is nothing but a certain kind of social otherness involved in them. Or, again, the "coldness" of green, the "distance" of blue, the "aggressiveness" of red, embody modes of variation fully explicable only in terms of experience conceived as a social continuum.

4. The intrinsic natures of sensory qualities, and not merely the order and correlations in which they occur, express organic attitudes, or tend, of themselves, to incite modes of behavior; and these modes may be appropriate or useful, in relation to the physical circumstances generally accompanying the occurrence of the stimuli productive of the respective sensations. Thus, of all the colors blue is intrinsically the most appropriate to adapt the human organism to the principal objects in nature (the sky, distant objects, and bodies of water), which reflect the short wave-lengths perceived as blue.

5. The first appearance of a given quality at a certain stage in evolution is not a pure "emergence" (though it has an emergent aspect) of the quality, unrelated to the previous state of nature, but is intelligible in much the same fashion as the appearance of a new organ. A primitive quality of sensation may be conceived, such that the development of more specific qualities may be made intelligible as a true development, or differentiation, rather than as a sheer displacement of the old and irruption of the new.

The acceptance, as a hypothesis, of these five theses in the organically interrelated form in which they constitute, as will be shown, one coherent theory makes possible a binding-together of the results of many distinct lines of inquiry, embracing pure geometry, aesthetics, everyday social experience, biology, metaphysics, and religious experience, into a sweeping generalization capable of manifold empirical verifications as well as applicable to the clarification of numerous philosophical paradoxes. The merits claimed for the theory, however, may all be summed up in one—that it opens the way to the observation and explanation of facts hitherto unobserved or supposed "inexplicable." The ultimate appeal is to the principle upon which all scientific progress depends: the employment of mathematical forms to aid in the observation and reduction to intelligible unity of the perceptual facts, guided by the one universally valid axiom so well formulated by Charles Peirce, "Do not block the path of experiential inquiry," together with its corollary, "No fact is to be supposed inexplicable."

If any other theory can lead the way to the conceptual unification of so great a range of observable facts, while successfully avoiding the baptizing of mysteries as "ultimate," of problems as "insoluble," of entities as "unanalyzable," "inexplicable," mere brute facts, then may that theory be preferred to the one hereinafter propounded. This may be summarily designated as the theory of the contents of sensation as forming an "affective continuum" of aesthetically meaningful, socially expressive, organically adaptive and evolving experience functions.

The designation "affective" for the whole continuum of experiences indicates that all qualitative contrasts, in whatever dimension, repeat recognizably the contrasts characteristic of affection in its typical cases, so that these contrasts may be said to generate the continuum. Such polarities are joy and sorrow, self and not-self, liking and disliking, etc.

The primacy of affection may also be expressed as follows: the clue to the observational detection of all relationships upon the continuum is the comparison of all entities thereon to those examples of affectivity which in psychology are most clearly and unanimously recognized as such. The doctrine of the dualism of sense and affection inhibits such comparison by asserting the incomparability of the two factors—a type of negative hypothesis which is the exact reverse of one scientifically fruitful or legitimate. If, therefore, anyone should fear that the word "affective" as extended to include sensation becomes thereby emptied of its usual meaning, this reference to observational signification ("operational," as the physicist would say) may serve as the answer. I am content to accept the verbally opposite doctrine, that affection is really a species of sensation, provided only that this be taken to mean equal abundance of observable analogies between the two, without denial or neglect of whatever facts and relationships have as yet been observed with regard to each. Granted the working hypothesis of continuity, and the observation of the facts, the rest is a matter of rhetoric only.

Another explanation which is required is that the "continuum" of sensory qualities is to be thought of as incomplete if it is actually occurring qualities which are in question. Complete continuity is probably never to be found except in the realm of pure possibility. In other words, there are certainly "holes" in the "solid" which might be formed of actually occurring qualities, but these holes represent qualities which in some possible arrangement of nature might at some time have occurred or may at some time yet occur. The empirical relevance of the conception of continuity in spite of holes lies not only in its enlightening us with regard to what may exist even though as yet unobserved by us, but also in the fact that measurement of degrees of difference can take place as it were over the holes. Thus I can find red to be more like certain trumpet notes than certain violin notes without experiencing intermediaries connecting red with the former or the latter notes.

### SECTION 3. THE PASSING OF MATERIALISM

The logical alternative to the theory outlined in the preceding section consists, by definition, in the joint denial of the specified five theses, and in the concept of sensation obtained through this denial. The polemical portions of the discussion are accordingly to be directed against this concept. An important feature of the criticism is the presentation of evidence designed to show that the criticized concept is the close logical counterpart, in psychology and philosophy, of the view which in physics is known as "materialism"; and which of late has practically been driven out of physics. It is my belief that physical materialism is a species of the same genus of doctrines to which the reigning theories of sensation belong, and, furthermore, that the objections which the physical form of materialism has encountered are only specific variations upon more general critical considerations which will prove equally fatal to all the species of the genus.

By "materialism" we shall not, in this book, intend the extreme and at no time generally accepted doctrine that all things are purely material or physical; but rather the far commoner and more plausible supposition that matter, in what may be called the "bad" sense, exists. This "bad" signification of matter may be defined in terms of the five concepts introduced in the preceding section as follows:

1. A materialistic mode of being is "atomistic," that is to say, involves radical discontinuity. The classical atom, both in science and in philosophy, represented a quasi-complete break in the texture of the world, and this in two senses. There was: (*a*) complete disparateness of quality between an atom and the empty space surrounding it, and (*b*) complete distinctness in being between one atom and another. In other words, absolute heterogeneity and absolute externality of relationships—the independence of a thing from its context—were asserted, or at least not clearly denied. In these respects sensory theory has until recently presented, and in some features still presents, a definitely materialistic character. The notion of sense qualities as "simple," and so unanalyzable, is atomism applied to psychology, and it was formerly the fashion to defend the notion on that very ground.

It must not, however, be inferred that a non-materialistic theory will be one that rejects every form of atomism. Such a theory will have, in the fact of human individuality and in the discontinuities everywhere manifest in experience, quite as much reason as materialism for denying mere undifferentiated continuity. But the atomic separateness so grounded will be a relative affair, more in some cases, less in others, and nowhere sheer, absolute separateness. Again, the reference to external relations might be taken to mean that antimaterialism involves the complete denial of such relations. On the contrary, materialism, in its usual deterministic form at least, denies external relations just where a truly spiritual philosophy asserts them, namely, in regard to the future, and hence to the problem of freedom. Also logicians have definitely proved that universals, at least, must involve alternate possibilities in such fashion that not all of their relations can be internal,[4] so that the absolute organicism with which idealists opposed the absolute atomism of materialists overshot the mark, indeed committed the same fallacy of non-relative thought characteristic of the Newtonian period. It has been hard to overcome the prescientific prejudice that the crowning act of thought is to assert and deny, to classify, rather than, as scientific method in its successful phases implies, to estimate or measure, and to elicit geometrical order. The hypothesis which all the parties to the debate over relations started by Bradley failed to consider was that internality is a quantitative affair, and that its maxima and minima define the two logical types of the actual individual and the most comprehensive universal, with the future included among the intermediate cases, and the present and past constituting the realm of the individual.[5]

2. Material being has generally been regarded in modern times as that which, in itself, or in so far as no other mode of being is added to it, is lifeless. "Dead matter" and just plain or mere matter have thus appeared as the same. Now, although a definition of life has often been thought impossible, I suggest that a partial explanation of this concept may be given in terms

[4] See C. I. Lewis, "Facts, Systems, and the Unity of the World," *Journal of Philosophy*, XX, 141–51.

[5] I have discussed these problems, *ibid.*, XXIX, 457–67, and in the *Monist*, January, 1933, pp. 43–50. See also below, secs. 4, 10, 22, 28, 34, 36, 38, 39.

of value. For when we regard a thing as "dead," we regard it as interesting, if at all, only to ourselves, or to some being other than the thing itself, whereas when we look upon it as alive, we feel at least a germ of sympathy for it; that is, we imagine ourselves feelingly in its place, we wonder as to its pleasures and pains, desires or interests. In short, besides being interesting to others, the thing presents itself as interesting, or something analogous, to itself. This is the only vivid unmistakable change, it seems to me, that occurs in our minds when a tiny speck under the microscope, for example, by a sudden motion convinces us that it is no speck, but a living creature. Now the physical atom was conceived as void of feeling; hence if there is a clear distinction between sensation and feeling, then sensation is the psychological counterpart of the atom.

3. The third of our cardinal ideas, that of essential sociality, is merely the union of the principle of feeling, conceived as the essence of being, with that of continuity. The latter is an abstract logical principle; that is to say, it is the form which existence assumes when regarded merely so far as relevant to the formulation of general rules of analysis. When existence is regarded from a more concrete, yet—if materialism is false— an equally general standpoint, the standpoint of life as value, the same feature reappears as the sensitiveness of life to life, of feeling to feeling. The sensitiveness is—again, if materialism is false—the fact of all facts, equally apparent whether one considers the relations of a man to himself, to his own moods, feelings, and memories, or of a man to other men or to a singing bird; and still discernible, albeit more obscurely, in the relations of a mathematician to his theorems or of a physicist to his electrons. The sense of participation in an objective cosmic intelligence which these latter relations, at least in many cases, consciously involve is not the only evidence for this assertion. A very distinguished physicist once surprised the writer by remarking: "The way to understand an electron is to sympathize with it." The spontaneous conviction of all exalted moments of life, which appears also to contain the basis of primitive magic, is the sense that love, which is to say, in its lowest terms,

the sensitiveness of living beings for each other, is the key to the nature of things. It is almost beyond belief how seldom learned persons can be brought to discuss the simple, plain question whether this ancient and almost universal conviction is true. Yet just this question and none other is the most general form assumed by the crisis in scientific logic which is upon us. If all things are organic to each other, and all are constituted of feeling, then the structural principle par excellence is certainly something strikingly like sympathetic rapport, which is the most generalized definition of love. Applied to the present problem, this question becomes: Are the qualities of sense modalities of sympathetic feeling and, if so, how?

4. Materialism may be defined in terms of its treatment of time. A thing may, on the one hand, be conceived as involving change in its being; or, on the other hand, change may be conceived as a series of entities or states each of which in itself involves no seriality or time. The latter conception is materialistic. Antimaterialism affirms that all being is process, that all change is activity of something whose nature it is to act; for since the change is essential or intrinsic, it is really self-change, or "action" in the proper sense. Consider once more the traditional physical atom. It entered into changes without in its inner nature becoming processional (it could be conceived "at an instant"). This is, of course, only another aspect of independence of context or discontinuity. This brings us to the fourth cardinal idea, which is that of sensation as essentially related to adaptive behavior. In psychology action means behavior, and there is but one kind of quality which, just in itself, suggests a particular mode of behavior, namely, feeling tone. Feeling alone is intrinsically an incitement to act, the direction of the action varying according as the feeling is pleasant or unpleasant, and perhaps in other ways. The physical atoms "acted" only in a sense in which their behavior and influence upon one another bore no necessary relation to their inner nature—which would not have been violated had they never been in motion at all. Just so, it is thought wholly adventitious to the inner essence of the datum, thunder crash, that it induces

the act of shrinking, to that of red that it produces restlessness, to that of sweetness that it produces the impulse to eat (at least in a greater degree, usually, than does bitterness or sourness). Here once more sensations are conceived as patterned after material atoms.

5. Since the atom was intrinsically timeless, it was of course not subject to growth or evolution. As for the sense qualities, these are usually admitted to have had, unlike the older atoms, a genesis, but it is not held, as a rule, that this genesis explains either the quality itself or its place in experience (why, for instance, the longer wave-lengths are seen as red rather than as blue), yet this is the important point. Inasmuch as the great factor in evolution is adaptive behavior, this aspect of sensory materialism is closely connected with the preceding.

The contemporary situation presents the striking fact that the first and the last two of the above-mentioned senses of materialism are no longer regarded as true of the physical world, while the two remaining senses are admitted to constitute, so far as this world is concerned, unverified and perhaps unverifiable hypotheses. For the first point, the relation between corpuscular units and surrounding fields of radiant energy is such that in abstraction from the circumambient process the corpuscles would, for physics, be equivalent to non-entity. Matter is dynamic and context-dependent, whatever else it may or may not be. The following quotation from an astronomer expresses the situation:

> If we ask into what ultimate parts the physicist divides the manifestations he studies, the answer is that he has never been able to make up his mind. He stands on his continuous leg till it is tired, and then he stands on his discontinuous leg, and sometimes he stands on both together..... The quantum phenomena demand an atomic limit, and the interference phenomena demand continuous waves..... On the whole, the peace of the truce seems to favor the continuous view.[6]

Need we go on to quote De Broglie,[7] C. G. Darwin,[8] and the rest? Analysis itself has become quantitative for the physicist,

[6] R. A. Sampson, *Science and Reality* (London: Ernest Benn Limited, 1928), p. 66. Reprinted by permission of the publishers.

[7] See *Cahiers de la nouvelle journée* (Paris), Vol. XV.

[8] *New Conceptions of Matter* (1931), pp. 209-21.

a matter of degree of localization, not of absolute presence and absence. This is the final triumph of the quantitative idea, and it is equally the destruction of materialism, the restoration of the logic, even if not the content, of true spiritualism. It should be added, however, that since universals may have external relations it is always possible to treat particles as identical in spite of changing relations. But this means that we consider certain slightly general aspects of the particle rather than its exact individual character. "Simple location" will always have a relative, but never more an absolute, truth. And as for qualitative diversity, who does not know that the distinction between particles and waves, between ether and space and matter, between heat, electricity and light, have become more and more deprived of absoluteness?

The tendency in psychology, too, is overwhelmingly in the same direction, as is shown by the emphasis upon "function," "the activity of the organism as a whole," "dynamic psychology," "Gestalt psychology," etc.

The second and third implications of the concept of matter, which like all its implications are in reality purely negative, constitute precisely the chief philosophical problem of the present. In physics the only authorized position in regard to this problem is an agnostic one. It could not be otherwise since, the data of physics being exclusively spatio-temporal magnitudes as such ("pointer-readings"), the only knowledge to which it can attain concerns solely the pattern of such magnitudes, the four-dimensional geometry which they reveal. Nevertheless this pattern, in the currently accepted form, is at least compatible with a denial of the two materialistic properties of lifelessness and non-social character, whereas the Newtonian pattern appeared to imply these properties. I refer here particularly to the current admission that determinism is at best a faith rather than a result of science, and to the rhythmic character of physical action. It is quite unnecessary to argue here that current physics gives more encouragement in detail to the Whiteheadian conception of events composed of aesthetic feeling as the materials of all nature than Newtonian physics could give to Leibnizian monadology. Either one does not know current physics and the philosophical conceptions in question or one can hardly fail to see what is meant.

But there is a further point. The appeal of the Newtonian scheme lay partly in the fact that it appeared so clearly imaginable. One pictured the bits of matter; one pictured their motions; all was clear. True, Berkeley shattered this illusion, and showed, if ever man showed anything, that the old physics was, so to say, only imagined to be imaginable, that in fact no one could possibly imagine a colorless, odorless, tasteless entity, neither hard nor soft to the touch, neither warm nor cold, etc., such as the Newtonian atom professed to be. Today it is certain of the physicists who insist that imaginative models will not do. A decisive reason for this lies in the inherence of time in the very spatiality of things. The old movable atom was really, even if unconsciously, imagined as palely clothed with sensory characters (visual, tactual, kinesthetic), though these were neglected in favor of its spatiality and motion. But to produce a similar illusion of an entity wholly independent of mental properties yet intrinsically a process is by no means so easy an imaginative feat. A vivid sense of something inherently temporal is realized only in the intuition of life, involving activity, purpose, memory, feeling, or the like.

The natural result is that the drift toward a frankly idealistic or hylozoistic conception of matter is one of the most characteristic philosophical tendencies current among physicists, and that positivism or agnosticism should be the most frequently adopted alternatives.

Peculiarly striking, though also highly puzzling, is the present status of the question of quality versus quantity. That it is impossible for quantity to exist without quality has been generally conceded since Berkeley, so that materialism in terms of these categories tends to have at most only a relative meaning. On the other hand, the inclusion of the "secondary" or sensory qualities in the concept of a physical thing has been found extraordinarily difficult to carry through consistently, even where the physical thing is conceived as nothing but a perceptum in the human or divine mind—a type of idealism whose popularity is distinctly and, in my judgment, deservedly on the wane. Yet if it is not the secondary qualities which form the concrete filling or content by virtue of which alone the geometrical concepts of physics can be accepted as adequate descriptions of reality, and not mere pieces of mathematical symbolism, what order of qualities then is it which fulfils this function? This is an as yet unanswered question, and we are told that physics cannot answer it.[9] Yet if experience is our guide, there is only one class of properties left for consideration —the neglected tertiary qualities. The Berkeleian advance toward the concrete whole of experience as the ultimate illustration of the nature of things may be proved to have stopped at an arbitrary mid-point which shares more in the disadvantages than in the advantages of the rejected extremes.

One of the reasons for the long reign of materialistic thought is that, since the power of reason is shown to perfection in the use of quantitative concepts, matter has appeared as the supremely intelligible mode of being, in contrast to the purely intuitive or "unanalyzable" character of qualities, at least of those regarded as simple. The "primary qualities" were those exhibiting rational structure. The quality of circularity as such involves logical relations; the quality of redness as such appears not to do so. Thus redness is of no real value as a principle of rational explanation. Moreover, it is not true that the relativity of "redness" to the percipient individual is matched by a relativity of the same order in shapes or motions as perceived.

[9] I am aware that certain species of "relativism" are among us, according to which this old-fashioned problem of primary and secondary qualities somehow vanishes. To me, however, it seems that the contention that "in relation to a perceiving organism" an object really has the secondary qualities which it is perceived to have is, as Lovejoy says, an irrelevant "truism" if the question is what physical things are *without*, or perhaps temporally *prior to*, percipients. "Objective relativism" may well be a true doctrine, but it is a very silly one if proposed as an answer to this question. The Berkeleian dilemma remains: either premental things had no secondary qualities, and then we must conceive a logically self-sufficient world as consisting of mere sizes and shapes and motions, mere relational patterns, or else the things were not premental. Surely we have a right to ask which, if any, of the secondary qualities we experience illustrate at least the general kind of quality premental things as such could have had. Does objective relativism really escape the fallacy of misplaced concreteness and at the same time provide an alternative to panpsychism?

For variations in the perception of shapes or motions are, at least in the main, logically deducible from geometrical optics, whereas we cannot by any means deduce either the normal "redness" or variations from it in any such perspicuous manner. We cannot—it is generally held—even prove what the actual differences in intuited color quality between one percipient and another really are, whereas if one man sees the saucer as round, the other as elliptical, it is possible to ascertain this. For these reasons the Berkeleian attempt to achieve a convincing representation of concrete reality by the mere restoration of the abstracted secondary qualities, without otherwise altering the conception of these so as to render them more intelligible, could not well have succeeded any better than it has done. The question arises whether what is needed is not a conception of the ultimate substance, "space-time," the "ether," the "mind," "being," or whatever you call it, which shall really integrate intelligible form with concrete or intuitive quality, as genuinely synthetized aspects of the final fact. That redness requires shape is intuitively evident, but the manner in which one shape differs from another appears to have nothing to do with the manner in which one color differs from another; neither in shape nor in color do we find a common principle explanatory of both of these modes of differentiation. Obviously space-time forms do not of themselves account for color variations, nor color variations for space-time distinctions. The real secret of the primary-secondary world is not revealed by these two classes of properties as traditionally conceived.

Only—to anticipate later discussions—in aesthetic and social notions of quality felt as that of a structure, a felt fusion of feelings into a whole, the same in principle whether that of a chord, a color harmony, a well-integrated personality, or a friendship, does the mutual relevance of things and relations become clarified.

The present situation is this. We are told, on the one hand, that physical reality cannot be imagined; and, on the other, that the sensory qualities by which we perceive and seek to imagine it, are "ineffable," "simple" entities, unintelligible to reason.

But there is a form of imagination here omitted from consideration, the sympathetic-social, and there is a form of sensuously presented intelligibility by which the highest functions and ideals of the human soul are experienced as "embodied," or somehow directly present, in the sounds of a voice, or the notes of a melody, or the hues and shapes of a picture. A psychologist of standing says of the ideal content of a work of art:

> It is not behind, we directly intuit it in the appearance. We do not hear tones, which someone has well put together in order to say this and that—we hear Mozart. (Busoni, in ecstasy, heard the bit of heaven that Mozart bore in himself. *Heard*, not inferred it.)[10]

Whether or not this statement represents theory or fact can be determined only by a careful examination of aesthetic experience. Philosophers and psychologists have too frequently adopted, apart from such an examination, a theory of sensation which prejudged its outcome.

The essential question is whether there exists, or can be created, a method by which such "spiritual" experiences, which are yet nothing if not sensuous or physical, can be made amenable to scientific analysis. As materialism was in the main only the shadow of our preoccupation with mechanical technology, for which things are *means* (actual or potential) but not *ends*, so the successor of materialism can be established only by a technology which aims at the control and theoretical understanding of things as ends, that is to say, by an analysis of the aesthetic and social phases of experience.

### SECTION 4. QUALITIES AND THE NEW DOCTRINE OF ANALYSIS

Materialism overlooks, I have suggested, the internal relations involved in individuals, as absolute idealism overlooks the external relations involved in universals. Now there is a third problem which is perhaps the most subtle and frequently misunderstood of all. This is the problem of the absolutely determinate or "specific" quality, which is neither an individual

---

[10] See Erich M. von Hornbostel, "Die Einheit der Sinne," *Melos: Zeitschrift für Musik*, IV, 295.

thing nor a general class of characters, e.g., "this particular shade and hue and saturation of red which I now see." Such a quality Mr. Santayana terms an "essence," and says of it:

> The principle of essence . . . . is identity. . . . . Every essence is perfectly individual. There can be no question in the realm of essence of mistaken identity, vagueness. . . . . This inalienable individuality of each essence renders it a universal; for being perfectly self-contained and real only by virtue of its intrinsic character, it contains no reference to any setting in space or time. . . . . Therefore, it may be repeated or reviewed any number of times.[11]

The Hegelian flavor of this identification of opposites—individuality and universality—is striking. In fact, I make bold to say that it is as good an example of a self-contradictory doctrine as the master himself could afford us. The independence of particular contexts which constitutes universality is due to and implies vagueness; and, conversely, the perfect qualitative determinateness of individual existences is due to and implies the definiteness of their relations in space and time. There can be nothing that is both context-free and internally free from ambiguity. For this assertion I will give two out of several grounds.

First, if there were such a thing, then there could be no escape from Bradley's paradox of the infinite regress of relations. For the essence, being quite definite apart from its relations, would in receiving them receive nothing, but would only enter into the relation of having these relations, etc. The paradox vanishes—in spite of Bradley—if we admit that in receiving the relations, in becoming embodied, the relatively indeterminate universal acquires definiteness in respects in which, as merely universal, it is conceived as indeterminate, or, as W. E. Johnson says, "determin*able*." Thus "black" does not, in ordinary speech, mean any exactly determined quality but a range of qualities. It is a known fact, moreover, that black is dependent upon contrast, so that "pure black" means absolute darkness seen simultaneously with pure-white light. It is at least questionable if this requirement, taken with absolute strictness, can ever be fulfilled; but certainly it is clear that we do not ordinarily intend anything so exactly defined. Both rela-

[11] George Santayana, *The Realm of Essence* (London: Charles Scribner's Sons, 1928), p. 18. Reprinted by permission of the publishers.

tions and quality are left somewhat indefinite in the universal or essence "black." When, however, we speak of this or that black as entities actually given in particular experiences, it is a different matter. For here the quality is made definite by experience. But so, likewise, are the relations in space and time. And if it be objected that many of the latter are still not, or not distinctly, given, I reply that the definiteness of the experienced quality is also not absolute. It is the merest dogma when we are told that direct intuition of an essence reveals this latter with absolute clarity. Those who assert this dogma must then explain how vagueness enters into thought at all if immediacy knows nothing of it. But Mr. Santayana would have a further objection to our reasoning. The dependence of black upon contrast, that is to say upon context, is, he would say, a physical or psychological fact which does not affect the black as a pure essence. With such a pure essence, as such, we are, he evidently holds, somehow acquainted. Seeing no scintilla of evidence that this is so, I venture to say that the assertion is pure myth.

Second, the origin of this notion of determinate but contextless qualities lies in an inaccurate analysis of the observed facts. The internality to a quality of its neighboring qualities is usually so slight in effect (perhaps with no color, for instance, so great as with black) that the quality appears to us as the same, even if experienced or imagined in a different setting, as an electron is conceived to remain still an electron of the same type under varying (though not under all) circumstances. But this sameness is approximate or generic. It abstracts from the absolute specificity of the electron and considers only the applicability of universals with slightly indeterminate boundaries of meaning. The exact character of the electron is not physically determinable. Similarly, the exact color quality is not the subject of the perception of constancy through variation—upon which perception alone the idea of essence is based—but only that less completely determinate character which is "the color of all objects comparison of which with this one would reveal no noticeable difference in my color sensation." But comparison is not infallible, even if its subjects are directly given. To compare we must identify two objects as distinct and to do this is either to alternate between two foci of attention, in each of which one of the objects falls into the "fringe," or else to set up a simultaneous division of attention between the two—in short, to diffuse the focus, so that it becomes little better than the fringe. In either case there is fallibility; through incomplete attention to one or both of the elements, or else through the diminution of vividness involved in comparing a memory image of the one as fully attended to an instant before with the other as this instant fully perceived. There is, therefore, as in physics, no possibility of completely accurate comparison. That which above the threshold of comparative error appears as an absolutely determinate quality, invariant in the midst of altered relations, is indistinguishable from the semblance of uniformity which would be produced by slight variations upon a more or less incurably inattentive or diluted observation and memory.

It follows from the foregoing that no absolute difference between, say, redness, as a range of qualities extending from light pink to dark brown, from blue-purple to yellow-orange, and any "one" of the qualities in the range can be discerned by intuition, any more than an absolute line or point can be seen in a plane.[12] An "individual" essence in this sense is a mystery or problem, not a datum, unless by this datum we mean the one identifiable entity involved, namely, "the-particular-color-which-I-now-in-just-this-part-of-my-visual-field-perceive." This is certainly something individual, but only because it is made determinate through context, unique by the uniqueness of such context. All other uniqueness is baseless word-spinning so far as verificatory experience can show.

It is only another way of stating this result to say that the repeatable factors which analysis finds in things are not to be identified with their real parts or components, but rather with

---

[12] It is curious that Santayana speaks of the continuity of the essences without seeing this problem, i.e., that continuity is not an aggregate but a law of division, of determination, of the undivided and undetermined (Aristotle, Leibniz, Kant, Whitehead, Weyl, etc.).

more or less close conceptual approximations to the real parts.[13] The parts of a thing are the spatio-temporal portions into which it can be divided, as in my visual field here and now is the green of the trees, and there and now is the blue of the sky, or there and a moment ago the white of the clouds. The green which actually fills such a portion of my world is not the universal essence green; on the contrary, the latter is only a more or less inaccurate criterion of comparison of the contents of many such portions. In this sense it is true to say that analysis falsifies; but it is a perverse way of expressing approximation or vagueness to call it "distortion." The latter enters only if we identify determinable essences with determinate real parts, approximations with that at which they are aimed but cannot exactly attain to.

In regard to the non-component factors which analysis of concrete things thus distinguishes, the most important problem for our purposes is whether these factors are themselves in all cases subject to analysis, or whether analysis is essentially of the complex into the simple. Granting that the terms of analysis are not components of concrete things, may they not nevertheless be components of abstractions, in such fashion that there must be abstractions which are the ultimate components of which all others are composed but which themselves have no composition and are therefore unanalyzable? In the light of what has already been said, this hypothesis should be regarded with suspicion. And it seems, in fact, to be a view altogether out of touch with contemporary knowledge. A competent logician, C. I. Lewis, asserts categorically that "logical analysis is not dissection."[14] The view that it is so he characterizes as a "false metaphor," referring to the physical process of taking things to pieces, i.e., separating their spatio-temporal or real components. Of course such separation can be done in thought as well as manually, and can be considered as a kind of analysis.

---

[13] This seems to be the basis of G. F. Stout's contention that the qualities of a thing are no less individual than the thing itself, although such qualities are also embraced in the "not further analyzable unity" which is their corresponding universal. As usual the impossibility of analysis means that the right mode of analysis has not yet been found. See Stout's highly interesting essay in his *Studies* (New York, 1930), chap. xvii.

[14] *Mind and the World Order*, p. 82. The entire paragraph is relevant here.

But that it is not the only kind is now at last made clear in physics itself. A French writer thus summarizes the situation for the whole of the natural sciences:

> .... The physicists .... have come to realize that the granular conception of matter does not represent the whole of its reality......[15] Louis de Broglie attributes to matter a discrete structure, composed of ill-defined individualities, whose uncertain contours detach themselves like flowing shadows from the background of continuity.[16]
>
> .... The cell which can stand for the atom in biology should in its turn be considered as a privileged localization where the characteristic elementary phenomena of life are accomplished: but these cells, seen in their true significance, represent individualities with inexact limits...... They participate in their environments, and their environments participate in their activity; they are inseparable.[17]

Thus according to the "wave-packet" conception of the particle the whole which such particles constitute is, in another but genuine sense, a constituent of these particles. The "simplest" entities turn out to have their share in the complexity of the whole system. Thus, too, the geometrical point, for all its seeming simplicity, has been analyzed into a complex system of ideas by the Whiteheadian method of "extensive abstraction." The true metaphor would run thus: Every elementary part is an all-pervasive wave-packet, is the entire system into which it enters (in its main characters, not, in an abstract system, in all its details) drawn to a certain focus. Complexity is identified by the point of view to which it is relevant. Absolute simples would be entities which were simple from all points of view, and the arguments for their existence rest, I think, invariably upon the failure to consider this totality of possible viewpoints. A fine example is afforded by the so-called simple qualities of sense, such as the primary colors, the possibility of analyzing which has been denied by psychologists, with exceptions to be counted on the fingers of one hand, although a point of view is perfectly possible in terms of which the analysis may be effected.[18]

---

[15] Techoueyres, "Le continue et le discontinue en biologie," *Revue philosophique*, CXII, 106.

[16] *Ibid.*, p. 98.   [17] *Ibid.*, p. 106.   [18] See secs. 5F, 20, 32.

If there are no absolute simples, then there are no absolute unintelligibles. In any event the assumption of inexplicable ultimates seems repugnant to the faith of science that what is is at least partially intelligible. If there are any limits to the truth of this faith they seem irrelevant, since each advance of science indicates that they lie farther ahead than has previously, and usually with great confidence, been supposed, and since if this confidence had been still greater the advance might not have been made, a form of vindication in which let those delight who can. The only possible motive for the doctrine of inexplicables, besides the mere fact that science has not yet explained everything, is that one does not know any way to explain or analyze explanation except in terms which imply such ultimate barriers. But to rely on this difficulty begs the essential question and, as we have seen, overlooks the fact that other accounts of analysis than those which imply unanalyzable terms are possible, and are advocated in the best scientific and logical circles. When the concept of functional analysis has completely triumphed, as to all appearances it soon may, we shall wonder how men could have talked so glibly about "not further analyzable entities," could have failed to see that such an assertion is autobiographical or historical in significance, meaning, to be exact, "not further analyzable at a given date by a given person or persons."

A more difficult question concerns the possibility of objectivity in the analysis of qualities. Are not qualities as such private? Our logical authority, Professor Lewis, himself holds that qualia are ultimate for science, not indeed because they are simple, but because, although they may involve structures, they cannot be identified structurally. There is for Lewis one ultimate division, that between qualia and relations; namely, the former are not identifiable through human behavior, the latter are so identifiable. But perhaps this supposition of a complete severance of behavior and qualitative datum is only a last vestige of atomic absolutism. Such a "dissection" of experience may involve an exceptionally subtle form of the false metaphor in question. We must dwell upon this at some length.

It has been suggested above that the absolutely particular and determinate quality is that whose context is determinate. Now there are degrees of particularity, as of its converse generality, and there are reasons for supposing that degrees of independence from particular contexts are correlated with degrees of generality of quality. Thus "color" seems to posit relation to an eye of a certain somewhat closely defined type, and to light-rays between about 400 and 800 millimeters but not necessarily to a human rather than to a bird's eye, and not to a completely normal rather than to a partially color-blind eye, nor, again, to one wave-length between the limits specified rather than to another; whereas "red" determines the physical and physiological conditions more, and "sensory quality" less, narrowly.

Instead of supposing that there are any relations which are not constitutive of the particular qualities subject to them, should we not rather consider the hypothesis that the only difference among relations with reference to a given type of quality concerns the degree of generality required to release the quality from the relation? Somehow qualities must constitute particular actuality; they cannot do this if they merely enter into extrinsic relations, which themselves as extrinsic would be general, repeatable. The whole complex would be repeatable, common to many imaginable worlds as well as to this actual world. Otherwise put, there would be no way of distinguishing the actual from merely possible worlds, unless we reserve generality and external relatedness, particularity and internal relatedness, as the characteristics of possibility and actuality respectively.

Professor Lewis' problem is whether behavior patterns are intrinsic to qualities. Now certainly there is a high degree of independence of such qualities and patterns. There is no obvious way in which "red" always means a certain type of behavior. Yet this does not prove that red makes no characteristic difference to behavior, that it fits all modes of action exactly as well as do the other colors. On the one hand, red is something general. It can occur in widely different contexts. This shows that there are relational factors too specific to enter into redness in general, even though they may enter into some particular this-given-red. But on the other hand, if behavior modes are extrinsic to red, it can hardly be because they are too specific, for there are behavior modalities as general as anything we can conceive. At least, on Professor Lewis' own pragmatic assumption this must be so. Nor, on the other hand, can the ground be that behavior modes are too general, for there is an absolutely particular, non-repeatable action in which the organism is engaged at any one moment, and there are all degrees between such particularity and the widest generalities of conduct. Somewhere between these extremes red should find its appropriate behavior correlate.

It is, finally, interesting to note that Professor Lewis, in an appendix, suggests that qualities are essentially aesthetic. Now aesthetic experience has since Kant been admitted not to involve any overt behavior, or even the desire for such. It is non-purposive experience, and rests content with mere contemplation. Nevertheless, there is good reason to ascribe this non-behavioristic feature not to the total irrelevance of behavior modes, but to the balance of incipient impulses to act. This thesis, which has been very ably defended,[19] implies that the elements of aesthetic experience are differentiated with respect to behavior.

Far more than these remarks, and perhaps more than anything to be said in this book, would be required to justify a very confident answer to the question of the connection between relations and qualities.[20] But I have perhaps succeeded in showing that there is such a question, and that the prevailing answer to it is inadequately grounded. The important thing in such matters is to break up the crust of dogmas which stand between us and that discovery of the intelligibility of qualities toward which we ought, in faithfulness to the scientific vision, and in spite of all obstacles, to aspire.

[19] See I. A. Richards, C. K. Ogden, and James Wood, *The Foundations of Aesthetics* (1922).

[20] The question is further discussed in secs. 6A (last paragraph), 10, 19, 22, 28, 37-40.

# CHAPTER II

# AN UNSCIENTIFIC HYPOTHESIS

\*\*

*The usefulness of an abstraction is relative to its agreement with the facts and its inherent simplicity of structure.*

BIRKHOFF

\*\*

## SECTION 5. THE LOGICAL STRUCTURE OF THE CURRENT THEORY

### A. THE CRITERION OF SIMPLICITY

IT IS hardly a fair charge against the theory we are combating that it does not conform to the usual canons of a good scientific hypothesis; for the essence of the theory is its claim to represent an exceptional case among scientific problems, to deal in fact with objects incapable of scientific explanation except in a negative or unusually restricted sense. Nevertheless, it is worth while to attempt for once to measure the precise extent of this unscientific or ascientific, this anomalous, character, the precise degree to which the sensory qualities are held absolutely and inevitably to defeat the human desire rationally to understand as well as intuitively to know.

Any theory, even a theory that there can in a given sphere be no theory worthy of the name, is composed of abstractions. Now an abstraction in general is a way of dealing with a multitude of facts as constituting for certain purposes one fact. It is a mode of unification of experience. There are, accordingly, two dimensions along which the success of abstract formulations should be measured, namely, the extent and variety of the facts so reduced to one fact and the completeness or thoroughness of the unification. Only by an incurable dissatisfaction with formulas covering but a limited region of facts, or gathering them into the unity of a concept which is little more than a sweeping-together of diverse concepts without any conceived internal connection, does science progress. Now I hold that the current view of sensation is nothing more than a congeries of abstractions without conceptual unity (even—as we shall see presently—without thoroughgoing consistency) and that it fails to cover the range of facts that a well-founded theory of sensation could be made to cover. In this section we are concerned with the first point.

The lack of "inherent simplicity of structure" which renders the current theory of sensation an anomaly in the system of the sciences may be brought out by a list of the principal types of apparently irreducible complexity which the theory tolerates.

1. There is the "modal" division of sense qualities in accordance with the eleven or so classes of sense organs. Intelligible comparison of qualities is to be confined to qualities given by the same class of organs (although the latter, as physical structures, can with marked intelligibility be compared to organs of other classes). For this dictum, laid down by Helmholtz and slavishly followed ever since, no special critically evaluated evidence has, so far as I know, ever been given, its truth having been thought self-evident.[1]

2. Even within these classes or modes there is much unassimilated complexity. For instance, the color system is generally said to consist of certain perfectly distinct and incomparable elementary factors, the "primary" colors, each of which is just its unique self and can throw no light upon the nature of the others. The fact that these primary elements fall into a continuous order of graduated difference appears thus as a brute fact not intelligibly grounded in the nature of the entities so related. Thus color, the most coherently conceived of all the modes of sensation, remains nevertheless a mystery and a paradox, a continuum without intelligible generating principle.[2]

---

[1] Recently, however, a psychologist has written of Helmholtz' doctrine that it "should be abandoned on general principles, for the reason that it limits possible theories without a single fact for itself to stand upon. It is sheer dictum. Moreover, there is already some positive evidence against it" (John Nafe, "A Quantitative Theory of Feeling," *Journal of General Psychology*, 1929, p. 209).

[2] See subsec. C below.

3. The next "irreducible" complexity in sensory theory is that such comparison as is now permitted between different sensory classes is expressed in the doctrine of a plurality of "attributes," which are not only absolutely distinct from each other but also fail genuinely to mitigate the disunity of the classes. Similar as intense, a "red" and a "bitter" remain nevertheless wholly dissimilar as red and bitter. Evidence that there is something wrong here is found in the fact that the intensity of a color is, at least to some observers, the same thing as its "brightness." This suggests that qualitative specificity within one sense can depend upon a mode of variation universal to the senses, that attributes really explanatory of sensory quality are not only possible, but that one such is a fact.

4. The class of sensory qualities as a whole is contrasted with qualities of affective tone or "tertiary" qualities; or, if these latter are reckoned as sensory, they are held to constitute an absolutely distinct class of the qualities of sense.

5. The very definition of sensation refers to the physical organs conditioning this mode of experience. Yet what could be more heterogeneous than the qualities which are its immediate objects and those organs! Even if one is a panpsychist and holds that the particles composing the eye are essentially of the nature of experience or feeling, he still will perhaps not hold that this experience constituting the eye is the experience of red when redness is the color perceived, or that there is any intelligible community of quality between this experience which constitutes the inner reality of the eye and the redness.

6. A similar gulf subsists, of course, between the sensed quality and the physical stimulus acting upon the sensory organ. Long wave-lengths resemble neither red nor blue, nor one more than the other, and consequently that they are seen as red and not, in general, as blue is regarded as a complete mystery or a mere blind accident.

7. Sensory qualities are the data or "contents" of acts of perception or awareness; or they may be conceived as parts of which the mind or total consciousness is the whole. According to some, the contents of awareness are of a totally different na-

ture from the awareness itself. Obviously this means a total lack of inherent theoretical simplicity in regard to this relationship, a denial of intelligibility at this point.

Idealists, on the contrary, assert—if they assert anything—a community of nature between awareness and its contents. Only they fail generally to point out clearly wherein the community consists. Blue is, they say, a mental state or functioning, a bit of awareness, not simply an object of mind or awareness. But since blue is an utterly immediate object, perfectly open to direct inspection, and since mentality is its entire essence, we ought to be able very plainly to discern mentality in blue as perceived; we ought to be able to see blue as a peculiar fashion, or modality, of being aware. But idealists have so far signally failed in any intelligible way to actualize this implied possibility. Moreover, in this respect the great majority of thinkers, especially psychologists, have been idealists, i.e., they have held sense qualities to be psychic in nature, but have neglected the detailed implications of this generalization. Thus, for most purposes, the dualism of awareness and sense quality persists.

8. Many admit volitional activity or striving to be a distinct class of mental functioning. Is such a function totally other in nature than the sensory qualities? If so, here is the eighth major breakdown of theoretical simplification in the problem of mind.

9. There is a common-sense distinction between mental states, activities, or contents and the person who has, performs, or perceives them. What more disparate, in terms of this distinction, than a quality of personality and the quality of redness? Contemporary thought, on the whole, allots to this disparity the quasi-absolute character it has for common sense. (Yet the latter is not, after all, wholly averse to another conception, for it is not an uncommon experience to meet people who feel a sort of qualitative community between certain persons and certain colors, sounds, or even perfumes. Indeed, the color of skin, eyes, and hair, and the sound of the human voice, are probably so regarded from time to time by every human

being, quite apart from sophisticated theoretical grounds, or in spite of consciously held tenets to the contrary.)

10. There is, as we all quite inevitably believe, some act or function of mind whereby we are set in relation to beings akin to ourselves; in short, mind as we know it is somehow social. Sensation, however, appears, in its immediate contents, devoid of social character. There is a sensation of the sound of a friend's voice, but not directly a sensation of the friend. And the quality of the voice is not, except by association, social in character. Here again is a dualism: the social and the absolutely non-social. The interpretation of the social in terms of the purely private is disappearing in psychology,[3] but we face as a consequence an absolute barrier to understanding of the relation between the two factors, unless the apparently non-social functions can be shown to involve, after all, a kind of sociality.

11. Viewing sensory content as a whole, one sees that it is the sphere of the conscious clues to behavior—the springboard of action, as one may call it. Yet, as it is currently conceived, there is an absolute dualism between such contents and behavior. A color or taste is not of the nature of organic behavior, nor does it involve, in itself, the least tendency toward such behavior.

On the one hand, then, we have functions of consciousness which tend to "adapt" the organism to nature. The patterns of sensory qualities, their relations of repetition and variation (for instance, the habitual redness of the blush), obviously thus serve to adapt the animal; but, on the other hand, the intrinsic essence of sense qualities (the mere redness of red) is supposed to have no adaptive character whatever. Any other set of qualities, occurring with the same relations of repetition, variety, and correlation to physical and other non-sensuous factors, would answer, we are asked to believe, quite as well.

---

[3] A sociologist has well said that without social relations not only no human mind but also not even an animal mind could develop. If anyone doubts this, he can hardly have watched the growth of a kitten or a bird or any animal of whose mental operations we can have much conception.

Mind, then, is active in part, and in part (if sense qualities are mental) is totally inactive: again, a pure dualism.[4]

12. The current theory of sense experience is dualistic with respect to the factor of evolution. New organs and species develop more or less gradually; but new sensations "emerge" full blown, as by acts of special creation. The theory of sensation, alone, almost, of all current theories, is pre-Darwinian. This point can be maintained while admitting a truth in the concept of "emergence" as currently conceived. The denial that the history of the irruption of a new quality could entirely explain the quality is not incompatible with the belief that it would explain it partially. It is coming to be seen that every effect is of the nature of an emergent whose preceding causes can never absolutely account for it; but we do not on that account give up the search for causes. So the search for a genetic explanation of redness, bitterness, fragrance, or warmth should not be discouraged by the doctrine that when these qualities first appeared they were pure emergents. Emergence and pure emergence are far from the same thing; the latter, for all purposes of theoretical inquiry, is, I must insist, pre-Darwinian. It is merely a less imaginative version of the special creation doctrine, involving the same objectionable denial of any possibility of a genetic explanation.

Here, then, are twelve sins committed by contemporary theories of sensation against the ideal of theoretical simplicity. They may equally be taken as twelve violations of the maxim of continuity, which is the first of the five clauses in our positive thesis. Continuity has by Charles Peirce appropriately been called the "word of all modern science."[5]

So far, then, as there is any approach to agreement among philosophers and experimentalists concerning the nature of sense data, this agreement envisages the latter in terms strik-

[4] See sec. 38.

[5] He did not foresee the quantum theory; but his own doctrine that continuity involves more than mere actuality seems to imply that the actual is invariably the discontinuous. Continuity is fundamental in science because the latter deals with what is in terms of what might be, and because the "totality of what is possible in a given direction," or of a given type, is, according to Peirce, always a continuum.

ingly at variance with the usual criteria of sound theorizing.[6] So far is this the case that it is almost by courtesy that one may say that there exists such a thing as a recognized theory of the sensory qualities, that is to say, of the materials of all detailed knowledge. It seems more just to say that there is a remarkable absence of any such theory.

In so far, however, as there is an attempt to justify this anomalous position of the concept of sensation, we are confronted with a theory to the effect that no theory is possible. The proposed explanation of the facts is that the facts cannot be explained.

But apart from the questionablenss of an explanation which makes a merit of its almost complete failure to explain, there is a more particular reason for objecting to the admission of irreducible complexities in sensory theory. This is the almost universally admitted truth that all psychological factors, especially sensory, depend in the most intimate way upon the physics of the nervous system. Now, this physics presents, on the whole, a highly homogeneous picture in which irreducible or non-quantitative differences are not conspicuous. How can a homogeneous world of electrical units be the basis of an absolute diversity of qualities? Even if the relationship between mind and brain be unintelligible, it must not be self-contradictory; and I do not see that the assertion of intimate connectedness harmonizes with the admission of thoroughgoing homogeneities for the one and radical heterogeneities for the other.

If it be objected that physics owes its logical simplicity to its having abstracted from all but spatio-temporal characters, so that the unity of space-time was bound, in the end, to triumph over all mere dichotomies, then let us ask whether the unity of the mind, of experience as such, which philosophy and psychol-

[6] If this judgment seems too drastic, the reader may be interested to read Pikler's summary of his own similar and equally severe estimation of the "current theory" of sensation, as a "scientific scandal," "lacking in that unity which science everywhere strives to realize . . . . an unfruitful assemblage of facts wholly devoid of penetration," etc. (J. Pikler, *Schriften zur Anpassungstheorie des Empfindungsvorganges* [Leipzig, 1922], No. 4, pp. 76–78). By different paths this Budapest philosopher and physiologist has arrived at conclusions as radically at variance with the traditional psychology as are those presented in this book.

ogy must recognize as the form in which all our information upon any subject presents itself to us, is any less implicative of a final relativity of distinctions!

Such is the logical structure of the doctrine we oppose. The conclusion is that if simplicity is a valid ideal of scientific theory, then the philosophy and psychology of sensation is still in a primitive state with respect to its working hypotheses.[7] We may also mention here the reasonings which, in all ages, have disposed philosophers to regard any unmitigated dualisms or pluralisms as in principle self-contradictory. Certainly diversity, in some sense or senses, is a fact; so that the reduction of all things to a concept of sheer undifferentiated unity would be wholly impossible. But the "affective continuum" is precisely a differentiated unity, a creative source of genuine plurality and distinction; so that the issue between this conception and contemporary doctrines is between an effort to relate intelligibly the aspects of variety and of unity which the facts disclose, and a tendency to allow these two aspects to fall so far apart that little intellectual satisfaction, and perhaps, in comparison to what might be achieved, little fruitfulness in the further investigation and useful control of the phenomena, are the result. The issue is then that of mere or blind, versus intelligible, diversity.

### B. KNOWING, FEELING, AND WILLING

An attempt is sometimes made to reduce the confusing complexity of kinds of experience reviewed in the last section to a more manageable form by the conception of a small number, usually three, of "elements" or most fundamental phases of mind, under which the remaining classifications can be regarded as special cases or subdivisions. In particular the description of the fundamental traits of mind as "knowing," "feeling," and "willing" numbers many distinguished supporters. But there is one feature in the usual interpretation of this triad which is open to serious objection. This is that sensation, as the intuition of

---

[7] Whitehead has told us to "seek simplicity and then mistrust it"; but the second part of this injunction becomes relevant only when the first has been acted upon—hardly the case in doctrines of sensation.

sense qualities, is generally classed under "knowing." But the whole point and function of this last as a member of the triad is thereby destroyed. This function is to account for the fact of meaning or symbolic reference, as something more than the mere intuiting or having of data. Of course, in so far as we wish to emphasize that sense experience is a grasp of objects, and not merely a having of qualitative content, we must include it under "knowing." But if we distinguish sensation from sense perception, and if "knowing" is used in the sense of intuiting—and only if it is so used, is sensation (thus restricted) an instance of it—then "feeling" would be another instance, and the co-ordination of the three functions in the triad would be destroyed. Feeling (in the usual technical sense) and sensation are the two main forms of sheer intuition or having of qualities, willing is acting or striving with regard to them, knowing is using them as signs of something beyond themselves, as instances of a class or the like.

That this union of sense and feeling under the same head is the only scientific one was effectively shown by the analysis of Charles Peirce, who pointed out that the most decisive classifications in science are those based upon mathematical form, and that the common form of sensation and of feeling is given in the fact that both exhibit (relatively) unitary or "simple" qualities (redness, pleasure) whereas willing, or better "striving," is conspicuously dual (an "effort" is always sensed as correlative to a "resistance"), and whereas knowing or "meaning" is irreducibly triadic (sign, thing signified, larger mental context or "idea" to or for which it has this signification).[8]

If "sensations" and "feelings" are thus classed together under the head of sheer living through of qualities, then there is one further fact of note. Of these two terms only the latter, feeling, throws any light upon the relation of intuition to the elements of striving and of symbolic reference. (1) In feeling, "striving" is implicitly incarnate, that is, there is a manifest relevance of these two terms to each other which is utterly lacking in sensory qualities if these are not feelings. Now such mutual relevance,

[8] Charles S. Peirce, *Collected Papers* (Cambridge: Harvard University Press, 1931), Vol. I, Book III.

organic union, of all the "elements" is just the principle to which nearly all psychologists today at least nominally adhere. A more genuine adherence to this principle will rule out once and for all the distinction between feeling and sensation as modes of immediacy. Only as feeling is intuition intrinsically united with striving. (2) The third element, "meaning," is also incarnate in feeling, and in sensation only if sensation is a form of feeling. That is to say, there is, as we shall see, always a relatively subjective and a relatively objective portion of feeling in experience, the relation between these having, as I hold, the "social" form. This social form of the life of feeling is the element of meaning, of reference beyond, which is essential to "mind." The "you" is never a mere quality of "my" experience, but something which that quality reveals to me. Feeling, in so far as it is social, is "feeling *of* feeling." This *of* is the meaning relation.

Again, of all the terms, "striving," "knowing," "sensing," "feeling," only the last (as we shall see later) throws the least light upon the principles differentiating one intuited quality from another. The principle of qualitative differentiation is either a secret of the Deity or it is feeling.

The relation of meaning to striving, finally, is provided in the concept of purpose, which is a meaning willed or striven for, a striving acted upon by meaning. Is there any other way than this—comprising (1) feelings, as sheer direct values; (2) action, as the influence of feelings upon feelings, in principle feelings or values socially objectified for each other; and (3) purposive reference, passing beyond mere reactions or conflicts among values to identities of sharable values—is there any other way than this of avoiding rigid barriers between mental functions, while at the same time accepting the factual varieties of experience? Mathematical concepts are the only ones under the sun whose identity of meaning for different minds can be strictly verified; and though we may argue forever about the qualitative difference between pleasure, pain, and redness, yet that all of these are akin in their absence of explicit or emphasized duality of structure (whereas striving is as obviously dual as it is anything) is fairly manifest and above all is a statement definite in its meaning—or one which could be made so by a degree of care which would still leave ordinary classifications perpetual fountains of ambiguity and doubt.

The reason for the traditional inclusion of sensation under cognition instead of under feeling is not hard to discover. Of course, this classification is pragmatic: that is to say, "cognition" means whatever mental characters function most helpfully to furnish man with information concerning the physical world, or with understanding of purely logical truths, such as those of mathematics. Plainly, sensation and not feeling (as ordinarily conceived) is thus helpful. But if our purpose is to understand mind itself, then this classification is no longer pragmatic but hopelessly confusing and pernicious. The mind is not first and foremost a machine for delivering information to itself about the physical world; but, so far as it seeks information, it seeks it above all about itself and its social fellows, and, more fundamentally, it cares about itself and its social fellows. Classifications whose end is the mind's social and self-understanding —that is, psychological classifications—should not be modeled upon those whose real motive lies elsewhere.

The true classification is already indicated by the "ambiguity" which is often complained of in the word "feeling" as used in common speech. Feeling in this legitimately broad as well as popular sense means simple qualitative givenness, abstracting from conflict of experiential elements (striving, conation) and from that relation of meaning (cognition) whereby one element refers to another.

All three elements, of course, are always present and interbiended. All actual feeling is a qualitative sense of an interaction between the subject and something else; and all actual feeling is feeling "of" a state of affairs transcending and partially determining that feeling.[9] Now no immediate intuition can or need be more than this. The rest is a matter of inference, more

[9] This is sometimes denied of certain feelings, but only because we sometimes fail to distinguish between a state of our consciousness and a state of our body. The latter transcends the former but is always given in it. The finger is felt to hurt—this is a reference beyond "my" pain merely as mine. Cf. secs. 29, 30, 39.

or less conscious, from the given qualitative content to a more definite picture of the specified further state of affairs. The remaining distinctions which the facts require concern, first, the dimensions of sentient quality, and, second, the degree with which the reference to an external ground is rendered prominent in various types of sentience, least of all in vague diffuse griefs or joys, most of all in the feeling tonalities whose sharp objectification outside the body, and in definite regions of extra-bodily space, constitute the sensations of vision. Logically this scheme fits all the requirements (waiving for the moment the problem of dimensions) and encounters as sole difficulty not any a priori incompleteness in the conception of mind so formulated, but the fact that people normally, including most specialists, have not noticed the thoroughgoing analogies of quality relating internal emotional with external or, as alleged, neutral contents. As a matter of logical structure, however, all the advantage is with the doctrine which assumes that this appearance of sheer heterogeneity is due to a hasty or prejudiced examination of the facts.

### C. THE GEOMETRY OF COLOR

An excellent example of the incoherence of current sensory doctrine is found in the treatment of colors, which of all sense qualities are those which can be most readily observed and compared to one another. The account usually given of the color scale is the following. Some colors, at least, are simple, unanalyzable entities. Certain colors, such as red and orange, perceptibly resemble each other; others, such as red and yellow, or red and green, do not. All colors fall upon a solid continuum such that there are continuous transitions from any one to any other. Now this is equivalent to saying that there is a continuum upon which the three points $A$, $B$, and $C$ are so related to each other that $A$ is a finite distance from $B$, and $B$ is a finite distance from $C$, but $A$ and $C$ are an infinite distance from each other. Thus red is like (has a finite degree of unlikeness to) orange, and orange similarly is like yellow; but red and yellow are not alike at all (have an infinite degree of unlikeness separating them). Again, if two entities $A$ and $B$ are absolutely different, it is not possible for a third entity *C* to be still more different from either of them than they are from each other, and by the same token it is not possible for that third entity to be more widely "separated" from either of them than they are from each other on a continuum the whole meaning of position upon which lies just in more or less resemblance. Now green is farther from red than yellow, therefore it is less like red in some respect (this "some respect" is necessary because via blue and violet a different relationship obtains) than is yellow; therefore, yellow is not absolutely unlike red. How could continuously graduated difference become at some point not simply more but absolute difference?

To show that it is possible for two entities each to resemble the same third entity without resembling each other, a critic of our argument might reply by an example such as the following: Milk resembles a hen's egg (namely, in color), a hen's egg resembles a football (namely, in shape), but from these premises it does not follow that milk and a football are related either in shape or in color, but only that they share in the highly general common character of being extended in space (the milk by virtue of the inherent extendedness of color as such, the football by virtue of its shape). In similar fashion, the relations between red, orange, and yellow may be, and apparently often have been, conceived. Both red and yellow resemble orange, but in such totally distinct "respects" that the only resemblance thereby established between them is that both are colors, have the characters inherent in coloricity, if one may so speak.

It is in such fashion that we might attempt to interpret the disputed doctrine of the dual character of orange. This color would then be conceived in terms of two standards of quality, according to one of which it is akin to red, according to the other akin to yellow. What are these two aspects of orange which constitute its alleged duplicity? The only answer suggested by the tradition is that the factors in question are redness and yellowness. Orange is similar to red by virtue of its redness, to yellow by virtue of its yellowness. Truly a marvelous answer! For the only excuse in terms of verifiable fact, for speaking of the redness of orange, which in fact contains no iota of red in the strict sense, is its perceived resemblance to red; therefore, if we inquire, as in cases of resemblance we always should, similar in what respect, it is silly, the merest vicious circle, to reply, in respect to redness. "John is like Harry." "In what respect?" "In respect to the quality of John which we may call 'Johnness.'" "Surely you are joking!" However, suppose Harry were simply to contain John, to consist in fact, of John plus some other factor, $X$. Then the foregoing description of the similarity between John and Harry might be accepted. Now, does orange contain red, consist of red in the precise standard sense, plus another factor, sheer yellow? This view has often been held. But there is no fact upon which it can be based except the perceived redlikeness and yellowlikeness of orange. The attempt to discern in orange a pure composition of red and yellow, the original form of the doctrine of primary and secondary colors, has failed utterly to command universal assent. No fact unambiguously implies it, and to many the fact of the perceived unity of orange appears unambiguously to negate it. If, however, the logic of the situation is not the logic of mixture, what mode of analysis is in point? The abandonment of the mixture conception, without the attempt to arrive at any other —the present situation in a nutshell—is nothing but the cessation of thought upon the subject, the abandonment of inquiry. But there exists an alternative mode of analysis, well known in other contexts, and obviously relevant to the present one. I refer to analysis in terms of geometrical order.

From the mathematical standpoint, it is, in the first place, doubtful whether a continuum may be conceived as an aggregate of distinct individual entities. A point is now coming to be regarded not as an element composing the space continuum, but as an ideal limit of abstraction. Similarly, the color scale is not an aggregate of colors, but a qualitative unity in which there is no such thing as "green," if by this we mean a quality absolutely free of yellow or blue, a sheer point in the line from blue to yellow. Any actual hue which has a finite extent—that is to say, any actual hue—will exhibit internal diversity of hues to a sufficiently fine discrimination. At any rate, the contrary could never be demonstrated in experience, and therefore has no relevance to the color scale as an empirical concept. But if every hue has a finite extent of variation, then it is arbitrary where one hue is said to begin and another to end. What is not arbitrary is then just the whole continuum, and its potentially infinite diversity of hues, each of which is a mere area upon the whole, not an element out of which it is constructed. Colors are thus aspects of the one fact which is "color." It follows that the apparent absoluteness of the difference, say, between red and green is only apparent. The unity which every continuum presupposes must be present in both of these colors, and must be present as a likeness. For the generating principle of this continuum is solely the likeness relation. Why, then, do we not see this unity, this likeness? Suppose a man had never seen any colors but red and orange, and always the same shade of each, a good red and a very yellowish orange. Is it not likely that he would distinguish the two colors absolutely, and never see either the redness or the yellowishness of the orange? Is not the "redness" of the orange brought to our attention by the fact that orange is so much more like red than are most of the colors we know? On the other hand, a standard yellow, though nearer to red than green is, is not so much nearer proportionately as to attract attention to the redlikeness which, in comparison with green, it possesses. If, however, it be said that this only explains our not ordinarily noticing the redlikeness of green but not our inability to perceive it when we do attend to the question, the reply is that we are not, in fact, utterly unable to perceive it. This is one of the facts which is at present often contradicted, but which we shall seek to establish later.

We have already discussed the suggestion that the similarities of red and yellow to orange must involve a duality of respects. The suggestion was made as a way of showing how yellow and red, though connected by an intermediary, orange, could yet be totally unlike. We have seen, however, that such total unlikeness cannot obtain. Nevertheless the necessity for duality in modes of likeness remains, as can be seen from the reflection that if orange resembled red, yellow orange, yellow-

## PLATE I

### Cartesian Co-ordinates for Color

#### I

#### AN IMPOSSIBLE SYSTEM

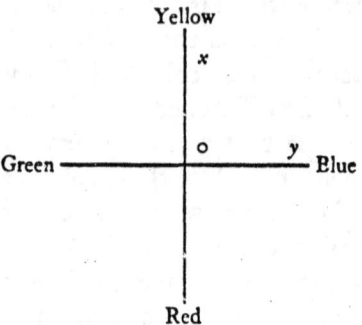

$x$ and $y$ cannot exist, since to order colors in this way is to contradict the facts. Yellow and red, blue and green, are not opposite extremes; nor to reach red from yellow is it necessary to pass through blue or green intermediaries; to reach green from blue to pass through red or yellow (in all cases avoiding gray).

#### II

#### A POSSIBLE SYSTEM

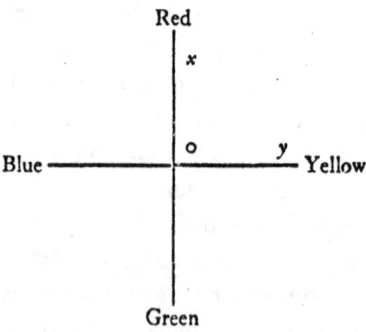

$x$ and $y$ must exist, since colors do exhibit this order. Yellow and blue, red and green, are opposites such that both extremes of one pair are intermediate or neutral with respect to the extremes of the other pair. There must be two respects of contrast in terms of which all color differences—apart from brightness—can be described.

green yellow, etc., all the way to violet, and all in the same respect, then violet would be the most unlike red of all the spectral colors, which is surely not true. Geometrically regarded, this absurdity corresponds to the impossibility of constructing a circular or self-returning linear order except in terms of at least two dimensions. The colors, abstracting for simplicity from contrasts of brightness, do form a self-returning or two-dimensional line. It follows that there are two fundamental respects of variation—a dimension being only such a respect—each of which involves its distinction of direction, that is, its contrasting extremes. Every place on the continuum is defined in terms of these two co-ordinates, with their four directions. No entity is any simpler, or any more complex, than any other, although an entity may happen to represent an extreme in a given direction. Thus, red may be the farthest "up" or "out," or whatever term serves to identify the given direction, along one co-ordinate, yellow along another, while orange represents a less extreme value along both co-ordinates. But red and yellow would then also, in another sense, represent medium values, each with respect to the co-ordinate maximally represented, in a given direction, by the other.

Similarly, all colors would involve the many-sidedness basic to the system, its duality of generating contrasts. No color could be one of these contrasts. The common quality pervading all reddish colors would accordingly not be redness; for redness represents a determinate value with respect to two contrasts, while the "reddishness" common to purple and orange, on the contrary, admits of wide variations along both contrasts or dimensions. If red is the maximum positive value of a contrast $W$, then reddish colors are all those with a value of this contrast slightly above medium, whatever value they may have in terms of the other contrast $H$. This quality of being a more than medium value of $W$, the quality of all "reddish" colors, is not the quality "red," for the characteristic of the latter is equally that it should represent only a medium value of $H$, the alternative contrast. This second condition is the least realized in yellow and blue, but perfectly realized in green.[10] Therefore, in this "respect," or in terms of the contrast $H$, green is more like red than yellow or blue. The latter, however, are more redlike in terms of $W$, since, being midvalues of this variable, they are not nearly so far from its maximum, red, as is the minimum, green. Yet yellow and blue, like green, are not reddish (possessing more than medium intensity of $W$). Thus redlikeness (lack of extreme difference from red with respect to at least one contrast, e.g., green), reddishness (lack of extreme difference from red with respect to both contrasts, e.g., orange, purple, brown), and redness itself are all three distinct. In the order given, each is a special case of the preceding. The doctrine of primary colors in all current forms blurs two or even all three of these distinctions and produces a logically unintelligible system.

What criticism of this general argumentation is to be expected? From experience I can answer: We shall be told that the use of a geometrical model is only a convenience and is binding upon us only so far as we have reason to regard its implications as applicable to the facts. Now certainly the use of a spatial model is merely illustrative, but the purely geometrical features of abstract order relations are what is here in question. One may employ any system of order relations one chooses to describe facts so long as that system is not self-contradictory. Now in the representation of the saturated colors as a self-returning line, square, or circle (all these terms in the sense of pure geometry), two sets of perfectly verifiable and generally conceded facts are symbolized, and (apart from details) beyond question correctly symbolized. The first set of facts is metrical. For instance, the minimum number of just noticeably distinct shades which can be interposed between red and blue simply is greater than the number between blue and violet. One may dispute as to the meaning of this fact in relation to the ideas of measurement and quantity—but the fact is unquestionable. The other set of facts is purely ordinal. For example, it simply is possible to proceed from red to yellow by just noticeable steps without

---

[10] The precise complementary of red is a bluish green. See sec. 32 for a discussion of the exact locus of the "primaries."

encountering hues of any other "primary" color than red and yellow themselves (and without passing through gray). It is not possible to connect red and green in this fashion without passing either through gray (including black and white under this term) or through one of the remaining primary colors, yellow and blue. These facts are as absolute as anything in physics.

Now the current interpretation of each of these two sets of facts involves inconsistencies. Distance, the metrical fact of the number of just noticeable differences between two colors, is in small values interpreted as degree of unlikeness, but in values larger than a certain quite finite amount, such as the less than one hundred distinctions between red and the yellowest orange, it becomes not large but sheer, absolute unlikeness (with respect to hue—the saturation might be absolutely the same, and the brightness would not be different by the amount of the distance covered). Thus yellow and green are equally incomparable with red, though by no means equally near it. The treatment of the ordinal fact of direction is no less capricious. In principle it symbolizes the mode or respect of likeness-difference between colors. Accordingly, change in this respect should appear as change in direction, as in passing from red to green via yellow. Yet it is supposed that there is also a change in respect in passing from red to green via gray, in spite of the representation of this passage as a straight line, implying, what the current doctrine of primaries denies, that red and green are polar opposites, extreme values, of one identical variable.

An additional inconsistency which is common in the textbooks, and which seems inexcusably careless, is the representation of the passage from red through saturated orange to yellow as a straight line, similarly the passage from yellow to green via lemon, etc., so that the circuit of saturated hues appears as a square. Since a square has its corner points farthest from the center point, and since the center point here is neutral gray, a square of colors means that the primaries are more saturated than the secondaries—a sheer falsehood, as Troland points out.[11] The only sense that can be derived from the square which is so

[11] See L. T. Troland, *Sensation*, pp. 355-56.

irritatingly aped from textbook to textbook (it is, to be sure, usually described as inadequate) is that the circuit of hues is a four-dimensional system, with saturation a badly represented fifth. But what psychologist has really accepted the responsibility of showing that red and yellow and green and blue and saturation are independent variables, so that we can alter the redness of an orange without affecting its yellowness or its saturation? However we regard primacy, nothing is known about it that can be represented by angles, except that feature which is equally representable by a circle (namely, that in getting from red to green through yellow there is a change of direction) and only the continuous or (roughly) circular change of direction will fit the facts of saturation. If it be objected that a circle has no privileged points, and that primary colors are such special factors, it seems sufficient to reply that in experienced space up and down and right and left are privileged directions, and if there were well-marked and constant finite limits in each of these directions they would constitute privileged points, but that this is no reason at all for holding that ceilings and walls must be pointed; any more than that the North Pole must be so. A circle can be described in Cartesian fashion by reference to two co-ordinates, the extremes of which hold a special place in the system without spoiling the circle. What defines the co-ordinates is another question, to be considered later (secs. 20, 32).

The conception of the color continuum as built partly out of similarity and partly out of sheer dissimilarity must be given up. Furthermore, if similarity in some degree, and according to the "distances" and "directions" involved, must obtain between all colors, then this similarity, though it may be unobserved, cannot be unobservable, for what is there to hide absolutely from us the basic similarity between immediately and very distinctly intuited contents? It is a merit in any theory that it leads to the observation of facts that are not otherwise observed. The current theory fails to lead to the observation of relationships which, as shown above, we know by inexorable inference from indubitable premisses to exist and to be observable. I submit that that theory will have established its superiority over the present one which does lead to the observation of these relationships, which enables us, for example, directly to perceive the similarity of green and red. Where continuous difference is perceivable, there is also perceivable the unity which makes that continuity possible.[12] If we do not see the unity, then we must somehow be seeing in the wrong way, and that theory is the right one which can indicate to us wherein our blindness is likely to consist. Let the champions of the *status quo* show us how, from the present theory, any such suggestion is to be derived!

### SECTION 6. THE FACTS

#### A. PAIN, TEMPERATURE, AND AFFECTION

If the inner complexity of the view under criticism were compensated for by a complete agreement with observable facts, one might perhaps seriously entertain the hypothesis that the phenomena of sensation are incapable of a logically satisfying explanation. But there are facts, not only of the writer's observation, but of common experience and recognition, which emphatically conflict with the implications of the theory, precisely in respect to its lack of simplicity.

First, we may instance a simple experiment which anyone may perform for himself and which seems immediately to demonstrate the falsity of two of the dualisms listed in the foregoing section. If one holds his hand in warm water, into which hot water is running, one experiences, of course, a transition from the sensation of warmth to that of heat. At the same time one also begins to experience a transition from a pleasant to a painful sensation. Now these two transitions are not given as sharply distinct, but, on the contrary, the intensification of the heat sensation and the more and more emphatic development of the painfulness appear as scarcely distinguishable changes. It is not merely that they occur simultaneously, but that as one compares the more vivid stages of the "hotness" with those of the "painfulness," one intuits a close affinity or near identity somewhat like that which obtains between red and orange.

[12] See secs. 20, 22, 32.

Heat passes into practically pure pain as orange into red—the relationship between them is perceptibly one of continuity. Similar remarks apply to "cold." We are not here stating a theory but reporting some observed facts.[13] Thus, qualities from two senses, one of them by all natural human conviction akin to the "tertiary" or affective factor of sense experience, have observably the same continuity of nature as qualities from one sense. This at one blow frees us from the dogma of incomparable modes and the dogma of incomparable tertiary, as contrasted with secondary, qualities. From henceforth these dogmas must be in retreat, retreat before the advancing array of stubbornly hostile facts.

The retreat might attempt, however, to call a halt behind a second line of defenses, as follows. Granting that pain is akin to temperature sensations—and recent investigations give scientific weight to this supposition—the gulf between feeling (pleasantness-unpleasantness) and sensation remains as profound as ever. For pain is not really a feeling of displeasure, as it seems to be, but a sensation plus a quite distinct factor of feeling.

> What we call pain is a certain sensation together with our revulsion from it..... Where the pain is extreme it is difficult for us to separate these analytically, and we tend therefore to think of the intolerableness as an essential quality of the sensation. In reality it is a comment made on the sensation by the emotional reaction to it; just as the beauty (or, for that matter, the pleasantness) of a colour or a sound is an emotional comment on it. In cases where the pain is slight we can abstain entirely from all reaction to it, and then observe that it is a quality of sensation, no different from hot or cold and simply more intense.[14]

---

[13] Recently, Pikler has shown how the sensations of touch may be combined with pain in a continuous system (*op. cit.*, pp. 62–63). Cf. also this remark by Burnett and Dallenbach (*American Journal of Psychology*, XXXVIII, 431): "Psychologically heat is a simple quality that lies in the pressure-prick-pain *continuum* [italics mine], near prick and closer to pressure than to pain." See also Lucile Knight, "The Integration of Warmth and Pain," *ibid.*, XXXIII, 587–90; and J. P. Nafe's summary of our present knowledge of temperature sensations in Murchison's *Foundations of Experimental Psychology* (Worcester, Mass., and London: Clark University Press, 1929), pp. 399–405.

[14] From C. A. Strong, *The Origin of Consciousness* (London: Macmillan & Co., 1918), pp. 315–16. By permission of The Macmillan Company, publishers.

From this and similar passages common in psychological writings we conclude: the very same logic, the very same type of evidence, which is held to show the disparity of sensation in general from feeling applies to the sensation of pain in particular, so that if pain can be altogether distinguished and analytically purified from affective tone, then doubtless all other sensations can be so distinguished, but if pain cannot be so distinguished, and if this can be proved, then the more general conclusion spoken of will have been demonstrated to rest upon a mode of reasoning which is unreliable, since it leads straight to a false conclusion in a certain test case.

It certainly seems clear that it will not be easy to convince mankind that the description of pain as a sense of evil contains no immediate or necessary truth, that for instance there might be beings somewhere in the universe who were so constructed that to them pain would seem precisely as pleasant as pleasure does to us, that it is only a peculiar human prejudice or "reaction" that connects pain with grief and unpleasantness, or opposes it to joy and satisfaction.

It must at once be granted that an emotional comment upon pain sensations, distinct from these, is a normal occurrence. And this emotional comment is not always negative or hostile. Pain can be positively enjoyed. These facts are compatible with the view of pain as itself a displeasure feeling, provided we admit the distinction between relatively objective and relatively subjective feelings. Pain is a displeasure feeling with a fairly definite localization, in cutaneous pain a localization near the surface of the body. It is thus a mean between feelings which seem to express the attitude of the self as a whole and those feelings which seem to inhere in a color or a sound outside the body in phenomenal space (see almost any writer on aesthetics, e.g., Volkelt). If one admits objective feelings, one must also give up the dictum that there can be only one feeling at a time in consciousness; for plainly emotional comments upon the emotional quality of a color or a sound do occur, as when one joyously notes the grief which seems to inhere in the whine of a suffering enemy, or in a bitter mood resents the joyous-sounding voices of those who are happy or the cheerful glow of the sunshine. The problem of objective feelings and of simultaneous plural feelings must be reserved for another chapter,[15] but some remarks may be offered here as suggestive of the conclusion that although pain can be enjoyed it may for all that be a displeasure feeling.

Who does not know that sorrow or grief can be delighted in and savored as though they were joy, that fear and horror can be sought and gloated over? Yet who, from these facts, would conclude that the feelings of grief, or of fear or of horror, belong on the positive rather than on the negative side of the emotional scale, or that they are not states of feeling at all? Is it not clear that it is their very affective negativity which becomes the basis for a superimposed emotion which is positive, as the sense of beauty is sometimes deepened by elements of discord genuinely felt as such? Who that enjoys a tragedy imagines that the grief of Lear in which by sympathy he participates is good and wish-fulfilling in the same sense as the enjoyment of the tragedy as a whole is so? In short, it is bad reasoning to take a paradox which results from the assumption that pain is affective as a disproof of that assumption, and as a reason for excluding pain from the affective realm, when it must be admitted that precisely that paradox, or something as yet not clearly distinguished from it, governs the affective realm throughout, is, as it were, a sort of little-understood law of the emotional life. As for the statement that a pain may be absolutely indifferent, I ask for an explanation of the manner in which such "absolute" negatives can be substantiated. After all, the failure to note any such feeling tone is not to be safely converted into the definite observation that none is present, unless it is assumed that introspection is capable of infinite accuracy (for given any degree of inaccuracy, given any margin of error however small, then a sufficiently slight feeling tone could remain undetected).

A second feature in the quoted argument is that if pain is affective only in much the same manner as any sensation, "a bad taste or smell, false tones, cold feet, etc.," is capable of so

[15] See chap. iv.

being, then the affectivity of pain is not intrinsic, since that of these sensations is not so. Now since it is just this asserted non-affective nature of sensations in general which we have found motives for calling in question, such an argumentation cannot appeal to us as conclusive for the non-affective character of pain; while, on the other hand, the analogy which the psychologist thus draws between pain and other sensations, when taken together with the insufficiency of the evidence urged against the common-sense view of pain as a feeling of evil (opposed to pleasure as a feeling of good), cannot but encourage us to endeavor to extend this common-sense view to other sensations to which common sense also sometimes seems to apply it, though perhaps in a more ambiguous fashion.

But if pain is essentially negative affection and if many sensations besides pain are also intrinsically negative in feeling tone, how is pain to be distinguished from these other sensations? To this the reply is that qualitatively there may not be any radical distinction. Certainly there are sounds which are strikingly painlike in character, e.g., the whine of a dog, or the shrieking and groaning of automobile brakes. Ordinarily, however, the word "pain" is used to refer to a sensation which has an intrabodily locus in phenomenal space, and this locus, together with differences in terms of other qualitative dimensions than the single one of pleasant-unpleasant, may well suffice to distinguish pain proper from negative sensations in general.

The intrabodily status of pain accounts for its greater tendency—as compared with the externalized sensations—to present itself as a mere "emotional comment" of the subject upon the stimulus. For the self is the life of the body, and the feelings in the body are hence the feelings of the self. The feelings intrinsic to external sensations are external feelings. Not belonging to the body, they do not, in a pregnant sense at least, belong to the self. They are object-qualifying, or not self-adhering affects, or, again, affects with "psychic distance." Now it is true that in being aware of feelings as belonging to the environment —or seeming so to belong—we tend to a certain extent to enter into them ourselves, to feel them as though they were our own.

Nevertheless a certain distance or freedom in their regard, a certain subordination of them to anything like the total or dominant feeling state is usually maintained. With this in mind, we see a further reason why pain seems to shift its status from that of a mere subjective feeling to that of a mere neutral sensation. For cutaneous pain at least is at the boundary between body and environment, self and not-self. Hence the interpretation of it easily shifts from a subjective to an objective point of view, and this, together with the prevalence of the dogma that all feeling is phenomenally subjective, might give rise to the notion of "neutral" pains, or pains that "do not hurt."

It is also not impossible to understand how a displeasure feeling can directly impart pleasure. A woman of intelligence to whom the question was put offered the explanation that in vivid pain one becomes intensely aware of one's existence as a conscious being, and in this awareness, "striking to the roots of the soul," there is a kind of thrill; and the same principle is expressed by a profound writer in the following words: "Tears"—that is to say sorrows—"are a wistful way of feeling oneself alive, and to feel oneself alive is always a kind of happiness."[16] The idea of pure evil thus probably has no meaning unless it be that of sheer nonexistence.

But if liking and disliking are not the tests of affective tone, what test can there be? Indeed, what meaning can this concept retain? Part, at least, of the answer is this: Imagine, or by experimentally controlled conditions cause, the quality in question to occupy as large a portion of consciousness as possible. Thus, if it is a pain, imagine the entire body to throb with a similar quality; if it is the taste of bitterness, imagine this sensation to invade, first the entire mouth, then larger sections of experience. Imagine or produce approximations to a state in which experience has become as little as possible more than a pain, a bitterness, a feeling of cold or intense heat, a sensation of blackness. If this experiment is really carried out, it will probably become clear that all of these states, in proportion as con-

---

[16] Dirk Coster, *The Living and the Lifeless*, trans. from the Dutch by Beatrice Hinkle (New York: Harcourt, Brace & Co., 1929), p. 80.

sciousness as a whole is assimilated to them, are given as affectively negative, as antivaluable, in distinction from either valuable or apparently neutral states. Pain can be liked, but only as a subservient, a rather minor, factor in awareness. Pain as a major, dominant factor is revealed as in itself a relatively inexplicit or unintellectualized dislike. Conversely, disliking, in its usually recognized form, differs from pain chiefly through its more explicit structure, its more judgmental character. The affective negativity of each is the aspect in common. If, on the other hand, the same procedure be brought to bear upon qualities intrinsically positive, such as sweetness, warmth, beauty of tone, fragrance, golden, the opposite result follows. If almost the whole of consciousness were a sweet taste, a fragrance, a soft yellow or golden, how delicious such states would be! They would doubtless not represent the maximum of affective value, for there would be a lack of contrast and variety; but in comparison with equal monotonies of bitterness, foulness, chill, heat, or blackness, the choice would, I am convinced, cause no hesitation to anyone whose imagination or whose experience really represents to him a vivid approximation to the states hypothecated. (How those whose thought is uniformly of the imageless type, whose imagination, in short, is atrophied, are to carry out the experiment, except in its non-imaginative form, I confess I do not see.) In other words, the total affective "spirit" of the moment may exist largely in spite of, or at least in contrast to, the spirit of a given portion of the presented content, the test of the spirit of the latter lying in the consequences of allowing it, so far as possible, to become itself the spirit of the whole. In this process, real or imagined, occurs a parting of the ways, whereby some contents classify themselves as intrinsically and in the main evil, and others as intrinsically and in the main good. This "in the main" is important, for pain need not be pure absolute negativity,[17] or pleasure sheer goodness—in fact, it is impossible that any value state should wholly escape the

---

[17] Cutaneous pain seems less purely evil than certain deep-lying pains (are these latter ever enjoyed?) and also than the less definitely localized feelings of unpleasantness. These worse negative affections, as we may call them, have, according to Nafe,

duality of aspects inherent in the Janus-faced concept of value. Perhaps all sweetness and no less all bitterness are bitter-sweet, with the difference only in the degree of emphasis with which one "pole" or the other is prominent. Even as a relatively totalized conscious state, bitterness might retain some good and sweetness some evil. Nevertheless, I believe hardly anyone could fail to perceive that in the first case the good, in the second, the evil, forms the less characteristic aspect of the situation. The good of bitterness is in conflict with its main tendency, and likewise the distastefulness of sweetness.

I conclude: The prima facie negative affectivity of pain, which scientific analysis has seemed to show an illusion, is reestablished by more careful analysis. The very fact that, in proportion as pain is intense, "it is difficult for us to separate" the emotion (the "intolerableness") and the sensation "analytically" is strong if not incontrovertible evidence that the sensation and the emotion are closely akin in quality. "Resemblance," says an eminent logician, "means the possibility of confusion."[18] The more readily two things are confused with each other the more alike they are. The orthodox theory of sensation plays a strange trick upon us. It demonstrates entities to be dissimilar by refusing to accept the only evidences for similarity which this relation logically admits. The business of analysis is certainly in part the discovery of distinctions overlooked by ordinary intuition; but the very fact that they are so overlooked is warning once and for all that the distinctions will prove to be somewhat "fine" ones, modifying but not negating the prima facie resemblance. This is all the more relevant where the confusion occurs particularly when the entities confused are vividly experienced.

It is true that we can distinguish pain from disagreeableness in general, for pain is a highly specific disagreeableness, but this specificity involves chiefly a peculiarly definite localization and

---

a certain dulness or darkness which contrasts with the brightness of cutaneous pain. As bright the latter is actually akin to pleasantness. That this is a serious objection to the position taken in this section is to be admitted. See secs. 15, 40D.

[18] C. I. Lewis, *Mind and the World Order* (New York, 1929), p. 364 n.

objectification of the feeling in a definite part of the body—or even, as with a man whose leg has been amputated, out of the body. Were pain really in itself affectively neutral, then the possibility of confusing it with displeasure, in cases where it is felt as unpleasant, ought to be matched by a similar possibility of confusing it with delight, in cases where it is felt as delightful. But this confusion has not been reported. Pain can be intuited as one in essence with true suffering, it can be intuited as "accompanied by" a sense of delight, but it cannot be intuited as one in essence with delight or pleasure. All these facts are compatible with the doctrine that pain is a certain species of true suffering, and on the whole they are not compatible with any other doctrine.

Thus the too great separation of sensation and affection has produced a no-man's land of pain in which the injustice done to both the separated elements is avenged by the impossibility of understanding, in terms of either element, this residual phenomenon. It is interesting to speculate upon the possibility of setting up schools of pain training, whereby subjects are conditioned to respond pleasurably to pain, so that anesthetics would become superfluous and physical suffering as such not only lose its terrors but become a source of inexhaustible delight. This would have few practical drawbacks, since, after all, mature persons could avoid the dangers of which pains may be the signs without suffering from these pains, as red may be understood to mean danger without being felt as dangerous in itself.

If pain is a sensation and yet, as I believe every psychologist in the world would, under the relevant experimental conditions —that is to say, upon the rack!—admit, also a feeling, and if there is no sharp distinction between pain and the temperature sense, and if in general the alleged gulf between sense and feeling derives from the same type of evidence as that falsely employed to separate pain and feeling, then the whole system of discontinuous classes, together with its corollary of the "ineffability" of sensations, begins to crumble before our eyes.

The truth of the foregoing is unconsciously conceded by all mankind, as is witnessed by those remarkably all-pervasive "metaphors," which are in fact some of the directest expressions in language of observed characteristics and real relationships of the "immediate data" which philosophers have so ingeniously sought to characterize in accordance with the emptiness, the unintelligibility, or "ineffable" and "ultimate" character, of their own traditional abstractions. Let us consider an example of this linguistic or literary deposit of experience, which differs from etymological indications of truth in that it is not peculiar either to any one language or even to any one family of languages, but is the sort of stuff of which all human speech and thought are composed. Universal literature is full of passages akin, for the present purposes, to the following:

> Woe unto them that call evil good, and good evil; that put darkness for light, and light for darkness; that put bitter for sweet, and sweet for bitter!
> —Isaiah

In this passage there is reference to a polarity common to the various senses and to the experiences of value. Consider now the assertion commonly made that though from the physical standpoint black is negative, consisting in the absence of light or of activity in the eye due to light, yet psychologically black is no less positive than white. If by negative is meant merely the logical negation of the positive, the sense in which "darkness" from the standpoint of physics is negative, then black as a datum is certainly a positive color, not simply a non-color. But if there is a kind of negativity of a real not merely logical sort, as evil, pain, and hatred are negative, and good, pleasure, and love positive, then for all men and languages black is the most negative of colors. Hatred, pain, evil—these are negative, for that which they negate or deny is none other than life itself; similarly, love, joy, good—these affirm life. Now black is physiologically a hole of inaction in a stimulated retina; hence in so far as the enjoyment of visual stimulation is a form of life, black is the negation of life, the abrupt thwarting of the will to live. And as such it is directly experienced. Those who do not see this are those in whom the habit of theoretical construction (they will at once talk of associations and other theoretical matters) is stronger than the habit of direct observation. If all this is true, then the correlation of black with physical darkness need not be the purely arbitrary affair it has been conceived as being.[19] This example is one out of myriads pointing away from the discontinuity association view and toward a genuine logical integration of the qualities of immediate experience, together with the physical factors conditioning them.

### B. PITCH AND BRIGHTNESS

There is one experience of intersensory resemblance which is peculiarly obvious to everyone. This is the intuiting of the "brightness" of high-pitched sounds. Moreover, since brightness is nothing but one of the three dimensions of the color system, the perception of the brightness of tones, if it can be taken at its face value, is simply the demonstration that so far at least as this dimension is concerned color and sound are qualitatively alike.[20]

A further common impression about sounds is that certain tones are "high" and others "low." Those psychologists who do not regard this phenomenon as inexplicable ascribe it to an association with the localization of the sounds, or the movements creating them, in the throat, head, or chest, in speaking or singing. Thus when I feel that the notes of the flute soar while those of the bass viol hover below them, I am unconsciously connecting these sounds with such anatomical experiences. Other objections apart, direct observation shows that this is not the true explanation. For what really happens is that one intuits in the quality of the low note or high note its lowness or highness; otherwise put, the spatial character is qualitative, not relational merely. This quality is perhaps best described as that of heaviness, with its opposite pole of lightness. Low notes are massive,

---

[19] Thus Locke, following Descartes, says: "Heat and cold, white and black .... are equally clear and positive ideas in the mind; though perhaps some of the causes which produce them are barely privations in those subjects from whence our senses derive those ideas" (*Essay*, Book II, chap. viii, sec. 2). This is a good example of the casual observations which have passed as facts in modern philosophy, and even, sometimes, in experimental psychology.

[20] On some supposed evidence that auditory brightness and pitch are distinct attributes see Appen. B.

dull, ponderous, and as it were earthy in tonality; high notes are thin, light, ethereal.[21] After all, colors also have apparent weight, and here certainly there is no bodily localization to explain the fact.[22] Even odors present the identical phenomenon. There are ethereal or "spiritual" and earthy or heavy odors. These examples suggest that we should resist the temptation to explain the downward tendency of low notes entirely by reference to their normally greater volume, for colors at least can differ in heaviness without difference in area; and, moreover, high notes can be made as voluminous as considerably lower ones if their loudness is sufficiently increased, without thereby losing their lightness, as is seen when many instruments play the same high note.

When two apparently quite distinct features are ascribed to the same qualitative variable, as brightness and elevation are to pitch, economy prescribes that we should look for some common principle connecting the two. A conventional view would be that once the "highness" was established (by association) then brightness would follow, inasmuch as the sky is brighter than the earth, etc., etc. But one who attends to the phenomenon of sound brightness will perceive that this impression is quite as direct as that of elevation or lightness. It is curious too that this very word "light" should ambiguously suggest both comparisons. And in fact, light colors have less "weight" than dark.[23] Is there any intrinsic qualitative reason for this, or must we accept the verdict: mere association? Now there is a perfectly definite test of the truth of the qualitative view. Namely, if

[21] Some recent experiments seem to show that sounds are heard as literally high or low in auditory space. "High tones are phenomenologically higher in space than low ones" (Carroll Pratt, *The Meaning of Music* [1931], p. 52). Thus my qualification "merely" was fortunate. But the problem is as acute as ever—why are rapid vibrations heard as up and slow ones as down? With color, location is determined by experience which has molded vision with reference to where colored objects really are. But high sounds are not, I take it, physically higher. The explanation I propose seems still in order.

[22] See Edward Bullough, "The Apparent Heaviness of Colors," *British Journal of Psychology*, II, 111 ff.

[23] C. D. Taylor, "Visual Perception versus Visual plus Kinaesthetic Perception in Judging Colored Weights," *Journal of General Psychology*, IV (1930), 229-46.

brightness is really a common feature of visual and auditory data, then the most decisive consequence should be that "high" sounds should be more intense, since bright colors (as painters say, colors in a "high key")[24] are intense in proportion to their brightness. If sound brightness is the same thing basically as color brightness, and if the latter is precisely color intensity (as many, though not all, psychologists hold),[25] then what can the former be but sound intensity? Moreover, this would explain the question of high and low. Intense energy is required to overcome the pull of gravity. It is the dead, the powerless, that sinks to the ground. All our metaphorical use of the vertical dimension emphasizes this, witness "aspiration," "low spirits," and the like.

But now we seem to have collided head-on with fact. For it is notorious that pitch and intensity—that is to say, "loudness" —of sounds are very far from the same thing. I reply—waiving physiological evidence to be considered presently—that the identification of sound intensity with loudness rests upon inadequate analysis, and that what there is of intensity, in the strict sense, in loudness is nothing but pitch. "What can this paradox mean?" you may object; "surely a sound can be made more intense ['louder'] without raising its pitch!" In answer I point to the fact that just as "brightness" is applied to sounds, so "loudness" is applied to colors, and as so applied it does not mean intensity alone. The brightest, most intense color possible will not make a necktie "loud," provided the area of the color is sufficiently small. It is a commonplace of color aesthetics that small bits of color are far less "loud" or violent than large patches. (In decorating a room, the general rule is the smaller the area of an object the brighter its color can safely be made.) In short, the strength of a color, in the sense of the extent to which it surpasses the threshold of bare noticeability and

---

[24] The word for visually bright in German, *hell*, originally meant auditionally high-pitched; so that the history of this word is the converse of our *bright* as applied to sounds.

[25] See Titchener, *A Text-book of Psychology* (New York, 1921), pp. 204–6, for an ingenious defense of the contrary view. See also sec. 32.

approaches the limit of its maximum possible violence, is a function not only of its qualitative intensity but also of its area. In color we distinguish sharply between strength or violence per unit of area (brightness) and strength due to the quantity of area. Now the chief difference between sounds and colors is the well-known difficulty in the case of the former of distinguishing between the quality and the volume of sounds. Sounds seem voluminous in a qualitative sense not true of colors. The reason seems to lie partly in the process of visual attention, the focusing process whereby we fixate and delimit one color area from another in a total visual field, the process being rendered all the more conscious by the eye movements usually involved. With sounds we generally attend to the sound mass as a whole, as a single entity. Yet there are exceptions. In listening to a softly playing orchestra at close range we have, I think, some tendency to judge the loudness chiefly by the quality of separate portions of the sounds. What with color is the rule with sounds is the exception. It follows that when we speak of strength (perceptibility) of a sound we habitually confuse or blur together two questions, strength of the sound due to its quality alone and strength due to the amount, the volume, of this quality. Nevertheless, the two questions can be separated, and when this is done the purely qualitative strength turns out (with qualifications to be mentioned presently) to coincide with pitch, as for colors it coincides (here also not quite unqualifiedly) with brightness. To see this in a general way we have only to consider the admitted fact that low sounds are voluminous, cannot be made as thin as high sounds can (by avoiding marked amplitude) be made. Suppose then a high and a low sound of barely audible and hence approximately equal loudness. Since the low sound is greater in volume yet no greater in total strength (loudness), it follows by strict necessity that its strength per unit of volume, its intensity in the narrow sense, is less. Low sounds, thus, are not merely large, they are inherently "diffuse"; just as high notes are not merely thin, but concentrated or "sharp."

When we think of the very highest notes, we do not, it is true, think of them as especially powerful; for the highest audible tones, being at the limit of the ear's range, are only one step from inaudibility—but this is because they are one step from imperceptible thinness. High notes vanish by approximating to a mere point, low notes by approximating to a mere atmosphere so diluted and impalpable that it becomes almost indistinguishable from empty space. (This would doubtless be more obvious if overtones, i.e., intense thin portions of the total tone, were removed.)

But we have still the fact that a sound of a given pitch can vary over a wide range of loudness. Is this, as our theory implies, a mere increase or decrease of volume? It is certainly in part that, as anyone can see by playing the same note loudly and softly. But there is at least one further factor, namely, the overtones of a note would also be increased in volume, therefore in perceptibility, so that the increase in strength is not quite so simple as it would be with pure tones.

It is doubtful, however, if volumic changes in fundamental and overtones are the only means of increasing loudness, pitch being held constant. For Halverson and others have found that the threshold of volumic changes is much larger than that for loudness,[26] and although the technique employed does not appear to have excluded overtones, it is another question if the difference between the limens is quantitatively explicable by reference to them. There remains one further possibility of explaining it without giving up our identification of pitch with qualitative intensity. Loudness is certainly proportional to area and average strength per unit of area—nothing else being a priori possible—but "average strength per unit of area" can have two meanings. Physiologically, the force of any stimulation depends upon (1) the average rate of pulsation of each nerve fiber (the strength of each pulsation being constant—the all or none law); (2) the number of active fibers. Now (2) may be increased in either of two ways: (*a*) by enlarging the area of stimulated fibers; (*b*) by stimulating a larger proportion of fibers

---

[26] See H. M. Halverson, "Tonal Volume," *American Journal of Psychology*, XXXV, 366 ff.

in each unit of area. Thus total force acting at a given time depends upon (1) temporal density, (2) spatial density, and (3) spatial extent of the stimulated fiber group. The second is called by Nafe simply "density," and is said by him to produce, at least in touch sensations, a conscious effect distinct from that of the intensity due to average frequency per stimulated fiber. He says: "Variations in density are .... ordinarily correlated with variation in intensity of stimulation, but we may set up conditions to increase density alone. If we stimulate with objects such as grills, a finer grill will be felt as 'denser' than a coarser one without necessarily any increase in other variable aspects of experience."[27] In vision, such an effect would not, to any marked degree, be possible, for the color experience is ordinarily completely dense, i.e., contains no holes whatever, and consequently the size and number of such holes cannot undergo alteration. This is due not only to the unique spatial sharpness of vision, but also to its related property of grasping its field of objects as a plenum, so that we do not experience absence of light as non-color but as the color black. In audition, on the contrary, silence is not as a rule anything but the absence of sound —though exactly how far this is true it is not easy to say, since there seems to be an experience of hearing the silence as one sees the darkness—and hence sounds may perhaps be regarded as capable of holes of varying sizes and numbers. On the other hand, in so far as auditory spatialization is relatively indefinite, it seems clear there would be a tendency for holes to be filled up by overflow, as it were, from surrounding active areas, so that intensity and not density changes would result from alteration in the holes. The rôle of auditory density, then, if there be such a thing,[28] is obscure; but when we have subtracted its contribution, if any, to the effect of loudness, true qualitative intensity or brightness must be the remainder.

[27] See John Nafe in Murchison, *op. cit.*, p. 395.

[28] Since these lines were written, auditory density has emerged as an experimental fact, no less definitely distinguishable than volume or pitch or loudness, in work done in the Harvard psychological laboratory by Dr. S. S. Stevens (to appear in the *Journal of Experimental Psychology*, 1934). Apparently this result is nowhere anticipated except in the foregoing pages.

The identification of this remainder with pitch constitutes the "intensity theory of pitch."

The primary variables of sound thus become:

> Loudness, or total strength, compounded of
> Qualitative strength, brightness, or pitch
> Quantitative strength or volume
> [Density or ratio of filled to empty areas]?
> Octave quality [tone color of pure tones?].

Secondary variables derived from the foregoing by combinations of tones[29] are:

Timbre or quality of colorful tonal complexes
Vowel quality or quality of colorless but approximately pitched complexes
Noise or quality of complexes both colorless and confusedly pitched.

The intensity-brightness theory of pitch explains many facts.[30] Thus, for instance, we understand the aesthetic characters of high and low notes, respectively, and the effects of ascending and descending the scale. The musical law of cadence —which is also a law of speech—calls for this and for no other explanation. Except under special circumstances we prefer to come to rest on a low note. Why if it is not that a low note is intrinsically more restful, i.e., less intense?[31] That very low notes are not used to close a composition is not inconsistent

---

[29] See sec. 33.

[30] Such a fact is that in "colored hearing," "the brightness of the color is determined by the pitch and [sic!] intensity of the sound" (R. H. Wheeler, *Readings in Psychology* [New York, 1930], p. 369). Also in Huber's very careful experiments the correlation of brightness with pitch showed "all the agreement that could be desired" (Kurt Huber, *Der Ausdruck musikalischer Elementarmotive* [Leipzig, 1923], pp. 128-30) between the various subjects. Huber concludes that "brightness" could be taken as a synonym for pitch, with one qualification—namely, tones rich in overtones are brighter (as pointed out by Stumpf). This exception perfectly proves the rule—for what does "rich in overtones" mean if not "composed of a large number of higher pitches"? It is interesting also that Stumpf, who more than almost any other psychologist gave his life to the psychology of hearing, seems finally to have adopted the view of pitch height as auditory brightness, after having earlier opposed it (just as he finally accepted Revesz' evidence for octave quality). See *Bericht über den 6. Kongress für experimentelle Psychologie*, p. 339. (Note Stumpf's use of "quantity of the tone" as identical with its volume.) For a similar statement see E. M. von Hornbostel in Bethe's *Handbuch der normalen und pathologischen Physiologie*, XI, Part I, 706-7.

[31] I owe this thought to R. M. Ogden, who however, indicates no relationship between the greater intensity of high sounds, which he here *ad hoc* concedes, and his general theory of auditory attributes (*Hearing* [London, 1924], p. 154).

with this assumption, for very dark colors are not so much restful as depressing—the diminution of intensity has reached an uncomfortable extreme. Again who does not see that a "piercing" shriek is qualitatively more intense than a groan could possibly be, even though the greater massiveness of the latter may render it quite as "loud"? And who, in the effort to imagine a sound of maximal intensity, would fail to imagine a sound both relatively high pitched and relatively massive? An example of such a powerful sound is a great siren whistle which may be both high and yet, for a high sound, relatively voluminous—or, better still, a large number of such sirens sounding in chorus, by which means volume can be indefinitely increased, until the intensity becomes unbearable.

I shall be told that "volume" in sounds is a totally different thing from volume or extendedness in the ordinary sense. But if it is a totally different thing, why should anyone desire, as almost everyone spontaneously does, to employ the same term for it? Moreover, there is too much mystery made about the idea of space, as though it were quite impossible to analyze the content of this idea and in terms of this analysis to determine scientifically whether or not a given phenomenon is extended in space. Leibniz long ago showed that space is nothing but the order of simultaneous coexistence, perceived as such. Where plurality is given as simultaneous, there space is given;[32] where space is given, there simultaneous plurality is given. Between the two ideas there is, apart from details (such as the question

---

[32] Banister makes the suggestion that the sense of auditory volume is probably merely the uncertainty with which sounds are localized. This seems putting the cart before the horse. If a thing seems to be at more than one point in space, it *ipso facto* as phenomenon has more than one part, one part for each spatial locus. Thus complexity of distinguishable parts is the key to the situation and this complexity is volume. See H. Banister, "Auditory Theory: A Criticism of Professor Boring's Hypothesis," *American Journal of Psychology*, XXXVIII, 436-40. Banister also mentions other grounds for denying volume to sounds, but these seem to me only to prove the vague and fluctuating character of tonal volume, not its unreality. Yet that volume is a supernumerary attribute is true enough in the sense that it is identical with that aspect of loudness which is additional to pitch (and density?). This identity explains such common speech usages as the following: "Some of the notes [of the hermit thrush] possess sufficient *volume* to be heard distinctly at a distance of a quarter of a mile." Volume is here, as often, taken as a synonym for loudness, a natural exaggeration of the truth that it is one of the two dimensions of loudness.

of why simultaneous order is three-dimensional), no discoverable difference. To ask whether sounds "really" have volume is therefore simply to ask whether they really have distinguishable parts.[33]

That chords, at least, may be given as simultaneously plural is beyond dispute. They are also never so "thin" as the thinnest single notes, and the more distinct the plurality the more definite is the spatial extendedness. Remembering that there are degrees of distinguishableness, we may, I think, unhesitatingly affirm that the more voluminous sounds are those in which a distinction between "this portion" and "that portion" of the sound (neither portion being before or after the other in time) can more manifestly and multifariously be made. Part of the sound seems here, part there, part still elsewhere—as is always at least vaguely the case where "parts" can be made out at all.

That area of colors varies with number of distinguishable parts, down to the least perceptible area, which is a speck at the threshold of visual resolving power, is apparent enough. Even the characteristic thinness of high sounds has its analogue in colors. A minimally visible area, well defined in color, can be smaller if the color is bright than it otherwise can be. A tiny speck is bright, a point of light, or it cannot be distinct in quality.[34]

It may, however, appear paradoxical that pitch, the essential quality of sound, should dissolve into mere intensity. I reply,

---

[33] Dimmick's subjects found "the volumic aspect .... as definite as intensity," and characterized it as "an impression of size," "total extensity," "number of elements" —thus confirming the philosophical analysis of volume as a totality or number of parts. Dimmick remarks that "no one has raised the question of the simplicity of the attribute of intensity," but does not himself achieve an effective formulation of this question, partly because he is less aware, apparently, than his subjects of the nature of spatiality (see F. L. Dimmick, "The Dependence of Auditory Experience upon Wave Amplitude," *American Journal of Psychology*, XLV [1933], 463-70).

For a convincing presentation of the evidence for auditory volume see Boring's well-known article, "Auditory Theory with Especial Reference to Intensity, Volume, and Localization," *ibid.*, XXXVII, No. 2 (1926), 157-88, esp. pp. 162-66. This was the article which led to the Wever-Bray experiment, to be discussed presently. It does not analyze the phenomenal nature of volume, nor of loudness, nor of pitch, and hence understates the case for the frequency theory of pitch which it defends.

[34] See L. T. Troland in Murchison, *op. cit.*, p. 185; and in the same volume, Selig Hecht, pp. 253 ff.

first, that it has not been proved that pure tones differ only in pitch height and volume, since "octave similarity" is not perhaps explicable solely in such terms. The series of tones may not, like that of the gray colors, form a straight line but a spiral (if octave quality has, as I suspect, two dimensions).[35] Yet even this is in part suggested by the visual analogy, for tones are responses to relatively homogeneous stimuli, and it is heterogeneous stimuli which produce grays! And colors could be arranged in a series of ascending brightness without calling upon grays.[36]

Psychologists are skeptical of analogies between the senses because some suggestions of this sort have proved deceptive. But the cure for hasty or uncritical unifications of phenomena under common principles is not to give up the search for such principles but to endeavor to improve the manner in which it is conducted. So long as analogies are officially banned by the doctrine of modalities, only casual, unsystematic, bootleg comparisons—that is, the reverse of critical and scientific—will be put forward. Also the very same absolutism which appears in the doctrine that modes are wholly incomparable will express itself in the notion that where they do have common attributes they must be wholly similar. Thus either sounds have spatial character or they are without it, as if spatialization could not have degrees of definiteness. Science is not the establishment but the measurement of likeness and difference. Unmeasured, unqualified comparisons can only discredit the attempt to compare. Perhaps this is the reason why no one except Hornbostel and perhaps a few others have taken the auditory-brightness "metaphor" seriously enough to have asked whether in fact high notes and bright colors were alike, and, if so, in what respect.[37] Yet discussions of auditory brightness are legion. If the intensity theory of pitch can be satisfactorily established, will this not furnish an indication of the unwisdom of despising

---

[35] See sec. 33.

[36] Whether or not there are auditory grays is discussed in sec. 33.

[37] However, Nafe notes the analogy of pitch brightness to brightness of cutaneous sensations, in connection with his discussion of the frequency theory of the latter (see "The Psychology of Felt Experience," *American Journal of Psychology*, XXXIX, 383).

the experiences of the race which are readily available in language? Common sense may err in over- or underestimating distinctions between things; but this principle holds universally: neither error can be more than one of degree. Where there seems to be likeness there cannot be mere difference; where there seems to be difference there cannot be mere likeness.

Let us suppose that the analogy of auditory to visual brightness had been taken seriously by psychologists, what would have been the result? At once the inference would have been drawn that a similar neural mechanism must underlie the two phenomena. This would from the beginning have told against the famous place theory as the *primary* explanation of pitch, since there is no indication of even the possibility of such a theory of visual brightness. Next, it must have been seen that place could not easily account for the relation of brightness to intensity. (This is not less true because we must admit it as a fact that pitches are localized in the cochlea.) That a place theory was ever seriously considered a sufficient explanation of pitch was a blunder of just the sort that has hampered psychological advance—a blunder of neglecting given facts so obvious that only specialists as such were oblivious of them. For, since visual brightness is plainly a matter of intensity of stimulus, and, as we know by direct impression as well as by easy and sure inference, also of response (why else should the middle of the spectrum be brighter than the two ends if not that the efficiency of the response shades off to zero at the latter?), and since auditory brightness is likewise a matter of subjective intensity, there was no appreciable room for doubt that the primary mechanism of pitch was a mechanism of intensive neural response. Third, this mechanism was set in a more definite light by Adrian's researches,[38] which showed a larger number of all-or-none responses with increased stimulation. From this moment on the proper hypothesis of pitch was that it was, at least in the main, a matter of neural frequency.

Meantime, the frequency theory had been entertained by

[38] See E. A. Adrian, *The Basis of Sensation* (Great Britain, 1928).

various psychologists, notably by Boring,[39] but not on the basis of the facts which made it a virtual certainty, like the virtual certainty of astronomical predictions of new planets, but upon purely indirect and somewhat inconclusive evidence. Boring was, however, sufficiently convinced and convincing to suggest and bring about a crucial experiment, the result of which, the famous Wever-Bray effect, seemed a striking confirmation of the frequency theory.[40] Action currents were detected in the auditory nerve of a cat which had the same frequency as the sound waves entering the cat's ear. Nevertheless, the great mystery and stumblingblock of a frequency theory was still to be removed, and it was this: How nerves, which in general have an upper frequency limit of less than one thousand pulses per second, could in the auditory nerve respond at frequencies of many thousands. The answer seemed to be a volley effect, whereby several nerves functioned as a unit, the unit having thus a potential frequency of the seven hundred or more pulses of which each nerve was capable multiplied by the number of nerves in the unit.

More recent tests indicate that up to nearly eight hundred pulses a straight frequency response obtains, that between eight hundred and at most thirty-two hundred an increasingly confused synchronization of response with stimulus, rather conclusively explicable as involving volleying, occurs, while above thirty-two hundred the only neural correlate of pitch seems to be place. What does this mean for our theory of pitch brightness? First, over about two-thirds of the piano keyboard, pitch is a matter of neural timing, and thus is a genuine analogue of visual brightness; second, over the remainder of the piano keyboard the increase in the neural correlate of brightness continues, but is gradually overcome by random, unsynchronized pulses, until finally at the top of the normal musical range, pitch increases are no longer the conscious clues to more rapid timing

---

[39] Boring, *op. cit.*

[40] E. G. Wever and C. W. Bray, "Present Possibilities for Auditory Theory," *Psychological Review*, XXXVII, 365 ff. A certain portion of the phenomenon is now known to have been an electrical artifact.

but become mere notations of neural locus.[41] Thus the brightness theory does not hold for very high pitches. This is, however, not a fatal defect in the theory, for it was arrived at as a theory of the normal primary facts of pitch experience, that is, as a theory of the pitches which we ordinarily think of as examples of the problem. The phenomenal fact is that very high pitches are felt as abnormal and queer, and that judgments about them become confused and difficult. In short, pitch differences at very high ranges are not values of the same variable as pitch differences at low ranges, and this fact is scarcely less well recognized than the facts upon which the brightness theory is based. That there seems to be some continuity in the mounting pitch experience, even after the thirty-two hundred limit, is open to explanation on the ground that the transition from the timing to the mere place mechanism is demonstrated to be gradual, since even in the lower pitch range an element of place consciousness enters[42] which, being gradually rendered more distinct, while the increase in the intensity consciousness becomes less and less perceptible, leaves no point where a mere ending of one series and a mere beginning of another can be registered. It is a marvelous mechanism for making two quite distinct principles of serial order appear to casual inspection as one.

What might seem a partial refutation of the brightness theory—the necessity to supplement it by a place theory—is really a demonstration of how useful it could have been. For the physiological facts favoring a place hypothesis were at all times so persuasive that there was never any danger justice would not be done to the rôle of auditory topography. The only danger was that the subservience of psychologists to physiology, especially to the physiology of a decade or two earlier, would enable the physiological advantages of the place theory to give it an altogether unwarranted predominance. Its rôle was doomed from the outset by undeniable even if neglected facts to be but a sub-

---

[41] See the report in *Science News Letter*, November 25, 1933, p. 339, of work done at Harvard by H. Davis, A. Forbes, and A. J. Derbyshire.

[42] The evidence for a place factor as well as a neural frequency factor in audition is persuasively set forth by E. G. Boring in *The Physical Dimensions of Consciousness*.

ordinate one. The primary fact of pitch is given as an intensive one, and with this fact all theorizing ought for the last seventy-five years to have been reckoning. The Wever-Bray experiment should have been made the moment mechanical and electrical means were available. How much saving of time this would have meant it would be interesting to know.

It is true that the foregoing account is an oversimplification. Visual brightness is not in a simple way a question of timing. To some extent it depends also upon the number of fibers activated; just as in audition the volley phenomenon means a complication of a similar kind. Perhaps the effect of auditory density has something to do with the random pulses coming in over the volley range. They do not enhance the frequency effect, but they do swell the number of pulses reaching the brain. In general, brightness is the correlate, not of any and every frequency, but of frequency in neural units that are too unified functionally to possess internal parts in consciousness. Given such parts, total frequency will be divided subjectively into brightness, volumic spread, and density, or the intensity of each functionally discriminated active unit and the number of units. But with all qualifications this seems an established fact, that in both visual and auditory brightness the brain is reacting to some form of neural frequency, whether frequency of single fiber responses, or frequency of responses in fiber groups. This is what we might expect from the all-or-none law and the phenomenal characteristics of brightness. A mere place theory could explain these characteristics only if we suppose that to place correspond also brain cells of enormously different sensitiveness, or else groups of brain cells of enormously different multitude, so that the quantitative factor demanded by the facts, and held by the pure place theory to be absent in the auditory afferent nerve, could be supplied by the brain.

An interesting additional confirmation of the quantitative character of brightness is the fact that nobody is blind or deaf to any part of the brightness range except the top or bottom. Tonal islands occur only above the point where the frequency response has begun to fail. Islands of visual brightness (which is not combined with place, but is pure frequency) do not occur. It is clear that while, with diminished efficiency, the higher frequencies might not be obtained, especially those requiring volleying, there is no ready way to conceive nerves unable to respond at frequencies intermediate between their upper and lower limits. By contrast, the place concept suggests at once the possibility of holes, inactive places. We have to face, after a century of evasion, the general question: Are the distinctions of kind recognized between different phases of experience, such as vision and hearing, such as sensation and affection—are these distinctions the final word, or does the plain man, any man not psychologizing, betray a deeper insight when by employing the "metaphors" of speech he implies an underlying homogeneity of experience, such that sounds can really be "sweet" or that sounds, colors, feelings, and temperature sensations can all be "warm" or "bright"? Science rests upon the discovery of unity; it is therefore a paradox that the speech of untrained men should postulate far more radical unities of the mental life than scientific psychology as yet recognizes.

Wherever such common-sense comparisons exceed in this fashion the unity now conceded by science, I predict that psychological, based on physiological, homogeneities will sooner or later be revealed experimentally. Will it not be a pity if this hypothetical agreement between universal intuitions and physical facts emerges throughout as an unanticipated by-product of investigation, instead of serving—as on sound logic it should serve—as a suggestive clue stimulating and guiding from the outset the formulation of physiological theories and programs of research?[43]

[43] The difference this would make may be seen by considering Troland's view that there must be in the cortex six chemically distinct processes for the primary visual qualities of white, black, red, yellow, green, and blue, and so on for all the senses. Our view would be that two processes with polar opposites might furnish chroma (in spite of the fact that "sensory control" of these processes would be triadic; see sec. 32) and that brightness would be merely the frequency aspect of these processes; finally, that whatever explained brightness would cover pitch, and that in general the qualities of one sense are sufficiently akin to those of other senses to render the number of radically distinct processes required very much smaller than the number of so-called primary qualities. See Troland, *Psychophysiology*, I, 109–28.

A biologist, complaining of the influence of introspective associations upon biological concepts, says:

> It seems to be a local peculiarity of our own receptor organs which draws such a sharp distinction between heat light and actinic rays, between sound and mechanical vibrations. The comparative physiologist can easily imagine a human being so constructed that his classification of the qualities of sensations would be utterly different from our own.[44]

But the fact is that, constructed as we are, and by the introspective method, the same conclusion of the relativity of sense classifications can be reached, provided we reject the unscientific myth that absolute differences could be verified by experience, and also if "introspection" includes the race observations, the common sense we have referred to.[44]

#### C. FURTHER INTERSENSE ANALOGIES

When a poet wishes to describe sounds, he may use such an expression as "the silver needle notes of a fife."[45] Note that the "thinness" of fife notes is not the only ground of the comparison to a needle. A sharp object is not merely a thin one, e.g., a thread, but one with an extremity both thin and firm, i.e., strong, intense. Hence only high notes can be "sharp." But the comparison with "silver" leads still farther. The brightness of the fife notes, i.e., their intensity or high pitch, is not mere intensity, just as a bright color is not mere intensity. There is in both cases some quality other than this which is present in an intense degree. If the sound quality of which pitch is the intensity were utterly different from the color quality of which brightness is the intensity, it then could not be the case that the fife notes should seem so beautifully comparable to the appearance of silver. For the intuitive aptness of this comparison is far more complete than any single abstract factor of strength could explain. Were strength the only common trait involved, the diversity of the other factors would render this unique ground of the analogy so obvious it must long ago have been subject to clear analysis. Besides, one has only to perceive the

---

[44] See L. Hogben, "The Biological Analysis of Sensation," *Psyche*, XI (1931), 43.
[45] Joseph Auslander, *The Cyclops' Eye*.

likeness in question to see that it is not a mere matter of equal strength of otherwise indifferently diverse qualities. The directly perceived fact is a similarity in all basic respects between certain sounds and a flash of silvery color.

If brightness of colors is thus intensity in a sense which makes them intimately comparable to high sounds, how is it with intensity in other senses? Are all "sharp" sensations also bright? For instance, sharp pains, a keen sense of heat or cold—are these "brighter" than mild pains, mild temperature sensations? I find it so and predict that naïve persons subjected to non-leading questions, scientifically controlled, would confirm this. A keen pain or pleasure has much of the quality of light, in proportion to its qualitative intensity (i.e., intensity per unit of area or volume).[46]

If sounds are describable as colors, the reverse is no less true. "The moon a tinkle of ice in a cool blue glass."[47] But here a third sense is brought in—temperature. It is notable that both sounds and colors, not to mention emotions, are naturally relatable to coolness and warmth. But so are sensations of still other kinds. "There are hot perfumes and cold..... Lucy's gardenias seemed to fill his throat and lungs with a tropical and sultry sweetness."[48] Is warmth, like brightness, a genuine intersense notion? Can it, too, be given a generalized statement demonstrating that it is not exclusively a matter of temperature? Is there any reason to suppose that the orthodox view of mere association is a truer answer to this question than it proved to be to that of the elevation and brightness of sounds? We shall see later that the two questions are in fact interconnected.

[46] Nafe says: "Variations in the frequency of impulses are correlated .... with changes in felt intensity, which vary between the relatively weak or 'dull' experiences of the pressure type to the relatively strong, or 'bright,' or 'sharp' experiences of contact, pain, tickle" (J. P. Nafe in Murchison, *op. cit.*, p. 395). The identity, both physiological and introspective, of strong, bright, and sharp is here recognized. See also Hornbostel in Flueger's *Archive für gesamte Physiologie*, CCXXVII, 517 f.

[47] Auslander, *op. cit.*

[48] Aldous Huxley, *Point Counter Point* (New York, 1928), p. 170.

#### D. MODES AND FUSION

A further objection to the doctrine of modes is the fact that sensations from different senses frequently fuse, just as do those from one sense. This fusion is not even an exceptional phenomenon, but in a sense the universal rule. Bichowsky says:

> When two or more end-organs are stimulated together so that two or more separate pre-sensations ("the first conscious effects that can be traced to a stimulus of the sense-organs") might be expected, apparently in every case fusion of some sort takes place..... When two such incongruous stimuli (visual and tactual) occur the first effect on consciousness is .... that of a single fused pre-sensation partaking of the quality of both tactile and visual pre-sensation without spatial discrimination of its two components but with decided emotional tone.[49]

Now simple qualities which fuse, i.e., form a partial identity, are not wholly different in essence. Furthermore, as C. A. Strong well suggests, all experience involves such a fusion of elements from different senses; for several of the senses are invariably felt as qualifying the same general portion of space-time, in which there is by no means room for all such qualities if they all remain perfectly external to each other.[50] In hearing a musical concert the whole mind is filled with the glow of the electric lights, which render visual space something like a plenum of color qualities; but the auditory space, which is well occupied with sounds, is felt not as a quite different portion of reality but distinctly as about the same portion. This can only mean that there is a considerable degree of fusion. Nor is it at all impossible to observe such a process introspectively.

Such observations, as is well illustrated in the quotation from Bichowsky, show also that the clue to the affinities in question is found in feeling tone. To reject, as we must, the notion that the affinities do not really qualify the sense qualities themselves is at the same time to abandon the notion that the feeling tone is really extrinsic to sensation. And, even were this not so, the same evidence (of fusion and similarity) which overthrows the doctrine of modes confronts also the dogma of the heterogeneity of sense and feeling.[51]

---

[49] "The Mechanism of Consciousness," *American Journal of Psychology*, XXXVI, 592. Reprinted by permission of the editor.

[50] *Essays on the Natural Origin of the Mind* (New York, 1930), pp. 81-82.

[51] See sec. 22.

### E. SYNESTHESIA

The facts of intersense analogy have failed to receive due attention partly because they have frequently been classified under an ambiguous or question-begging caption, namely, as cases of "synesthesia," which is regarded as a phenomenon peculiar to certain persons. The general premiss upon which most discussions of "synesthetic" phenomena have been based is that the relationships experienced between two types of sense quality (such as sounds and colors, in so-called "colored hearing") concern merely the factual togetherness, association, or simultaneous production, of the two types, but by no possibility their qualitative similarity.[52] This premiss is derived from the general dogma of sensuous heterogeneity first expressed by Helmholtz and quoted in chapter i of this book. Upon what evidence did Helmholtz base this distinction between sensory modes, i.e., incomparable classes of sensory qualities? There seem to be four possible answers. First, and I believe this is the true answer, Helmholtz may have regarded the matter as entirely self-evident, as an intuitive axiom calling for no special justification or criticism. Second, he may have induced his conclusion from the empirical fact that the supposedly incomparable qualities are such as people do not attempt to compare. But in that case his fact was an invention; nothing is commoner than such comparisons (e.g., "bitter cold"). Third, he may have meant that psychologists have not discovered any well-attested similarities between qualities of different modes. This may have

---

[52] Lest I be thought to attack a straw man, I give an example. Burnett and Dallenbach report a subject as saying, "The warm and cold appeared gray .... there is nothing gray there, but that's the best way to describe the experience." And again, "Two temperature experiences that appeared as cold and warm pressures. Although *there is no visual stuff there* [italics mine], the experience can best be described as a large gray square which is rather dense .... at the top of which is a strip of gray smoke. ...." The authors conclude that these accounts represent not attempts to describe the difference between the various temperature sensations but rather assertions of simultaneous thermal and visual imagery—in short, "it is obvious that they [the phenomena] are synesthetic." Several reasons are given, every one of which seems to me a distortion of the protocols. What the subjects say is simply and clearly that the thermal sensations as such were like certain visual images (not present) in quality. In short, they support the doctrine of the comparability of different sensory modes and give no indication of synesthesia in the orthodox sense. See Burnett and Dallenbach, "The Experience of Heat," *Amer. Jour. of Psychol.*, XXXVIII, 430. Reprinted by permission of the editor.

been true; but of course it is dangerous to use such previous inability to discover such relations as evidence that there is nothing to discover. Fourth, Helmholtz may have felt that the distinctness of the organs underlying the sensory modes implied the complete disparity of the sensations depending on those organs. But in that case he was certainly mistaken. The nerve impulse from all the sense organs is now thought to be the same except for the number of impulses per unit of time and the number of fibers. The psychological correlate of this conception is certainly not the doctrine of modes in its traditional form. In short, we see that Helmholtz' axiom was an appeal to uncriticized self-evidence which is contradicted by the verdict of experience. Nevertheless, from this axiom has been derived the widespread assumption that synesthetic phenomena cannot possibly have anything to do with real similarities.[53]

But we must not exaggerate; there was one further ground for the same assumption. This was the apparent fact of the lack of consistency and of universality found to characterize synesthetic experiences. If there were genuinely objective affinities between sounds and colors, then everyone would experience them in fundamentally the same fashion; and this is notoriously not the case. Perhaps this assumption is self-evident? On the contrary, it is open to reasonable doubt. The objective truth of an analogy is not necessarily a sufficient guaranty that it will be observed; objective is not equivalent to obvious or readily detected and described. We observe chiefly what practical life has made important, and our ability to report in unambiguous terms what we have observed has many a limitation. In the instance before us these general considerations are strengthened by the special circumstances. Some of the subjects may have been partially tone deaf and so through missing some of the overtones received a decidedly altered timbre of sound; in some instances there may have been partial color-blindness. Very often, too, argument is made from such loose statements as that a certain instrument (presumably at any pitch) or a cer-

---

[53] A contrary assumption is sometimes met with, however, even in early investigations into the subject.

tain pitch (presumably on any instrument) is related to a certain color (presumably at any brightness and saturation). These are obviously vague generalizations, on the face of them devoid of precise meaning or truth. Still vaguer are likely to be the references to the color of vowels, where ocular, auditory, and other factors are exceptionally complicated and varied. But even if all these uncertainties have been sufficiently considered and controlled, the conclusion drawn of the hopeless disagreement of different subjects requires further justification. Let us consider an example from a much less difficult sphere. Suppose a very dull orange brown; required to determine whether the brown is closer to red or to yellow. Is it not possible that one subject should report the brown as a red brown, another as a yellow brown or tan, and still a third as an orange brown? Is there no difficulty in this sort of comparison? If there is at least some difficulty here, then we are justified in supposing there must be much more in accurately reporting upon any relations which may obtain between sounds and colors, where it is so easy to be confused by the differences between the ways in which we intuit the two types of data, the different functionings of the sense organs and indeed of the entire organism, and where there has yet been constructed no general scheme comparable to the system of colors by reference to which a "line" of similarity may be specified. Indeed, there is no adequate schematic representation of sounds by themselves.

In sum, the psychologist's procedure in respect to synesthesia has been about as follows. He was first struck by the broad fact of certain obvious similarity lines running through experience, dividing it naturally into certain classes roughly agreeing with the even more obvious classifications based upon the relations to a common or a different sense organ. Seeing no other similarity relationships of so obvious a character (either from the introspective or from the anatomical standpoints), and being preoccupied with the ideal—in itself sound, for this early stage of his science—of achieving neat divisions between phenomena, comparable to those which formerly obtained in physical science, he at once leaped to the conclusion, pronounced as a dogma, that the clean lines of this separation into classes could never be blurred by the discovery of cross-classifications,[54] by the discovery, for instance, that red is as truly "nearer" to certain sounds (say certain notes of the trumpet) than to green as it is nearer to orange than to green.

From the outset this doctrine of incomparability was contradicted by facts only slightly less manifest than those upon which it was founded. For instance, the experience of taste and smells, so far from teaching us the utter heterogeneity of these two modes, shows us that it is difficult at times to observe any difference between them. Will anyone maintain that sweetness as a taste quality has no closer affinity of essence with sweetness of smell than it has with a putrid odor? Are there not sourlike smells and bitter-like? What blind dogmatism to deny that in the eating of ice-cream the senses of taste, of cold, of smoothness, of smell, are all so interblended, and far indeed from absolutely heterogeneous, that it is not decided kinship but significant difference of quality that is hard to detect. It would be interesting to know what the tests of similarity are supposed to be by the defenders of the non-similarity of modes.[55]

When, however, certain persons, often those distinguished for their fine, accurate, and trained powers of sensory discrimination, have declared emphatically that to them sensations from different modes appeared very distinctly and indubitably comparable,[56] the psychologist has formed the suspicion that these persons were characterized by odd personal idiosyncrasies having no bearings upon any question of the real relationships of the sense qualities. This suspicion was encouraged at the outset by the psychologist's own lack of such experiences; strengthened almost immediately by the results of investigations appear-

[54] Cf. Pratt, *op. cit.*, pp. 179-80; and Wolfgang Köhler, *Gestalt Psychology*, pp. 241-42.

[55] E. M. von Hornbostel has a fine statement of the evidences for intersensory analogies in his "Die Einheit der Sinne," *Melos: Zeitschrift für Musik*, IV, 290-97.

[56] E.g., the composer Hoffman says, "It is not only in dreams, it is also when awake, when I hear some music, that I find an analogy and an intimate union between colors, sounds, and perfumes. It seems to me that all these things have been generated by some ray of light, and that they must be reunited in some wonderful harmony ...." (quoted in S. A. Rhodes, *The Cult of Beauty in Charles Baudelaire*, I, 145-46).

ing to establish conclusively: (1) that only a certain minority of persons are "synesthetic"; and (2) that these persons do not agree as to the particular relationships of qualities established by their experiences. Thus the subjective character of the phenomena, and consequently their incapacity to disturb the doctrine of modes, was apparently established. The unproved assumption, previously pointed out, of the identity of qualitative analogies which really obtain and those which are easy to detect and describe with accuracy passed unnoticed. That perhaps the chief difference between most "synesthetic" persons and others lies simply in the greater aptitude of the former to observe relationships which actually obtain in the experience of everyone—namely, relationships of similarity—was scarcely thought of even as an unlikely hypothesis. Yet this very explanation is the one offered spontaneously by some of the subjects. We are told that there was a tendency to insist that the colored hearing did not mean that when a sound was heard it was accompanied by an image of a certain color, but rather that the sound was found to be "like" the color.[57] It need not occasion surprise that this report was held of no consequence by the investigator, although it was honestly recorded by him. For if he had taken it seriously, he would have found himself doubting a fundamental tenet of psychology, and it is only in a less difficult science than psychology that a few facts are enough to overthrow a dogma. But there were, and are, more than a few facts. There was the fact, which has occasioned some amazement, that synesthetic persons insist with almost if not complete unanimity that what they see others must be able to see, that the colors and sounds which they find related are so related and that this should be apparent to anyone. Since such persons are often highly intelligent, it is a little strange that they should be unable to realize that a simultaneous excitation of two heterogeneous elements, or an association of the two, is logically arbitrary with respect to the elements and need by no means hold for others. But on the contrary we are told that they often insist

---

[57] See Charles Myers, "A Case of Synaesthesia," *British Journal of Psychology*, IV, 228 ff., and VII, 112 ff.

that similarity and not mere connection is the plain fact of the experience. Naturally, then, they cannot admit that others can be incapable of seeing it so, on the same basis as one would be surprised if someone could not see that a brown was reddish, if one clearly saw this affinity to red one's self. Nevertheless such likenesses can be overlooked or differently estimated.

Whether cases which conform to the formula of synesthesia as it has been construed—namely, as a sort of abnormal simultaneity of two different sense modalities where only one is stimulated—are also actual occurrences I do not know; but there appears good reason to suppose it. Some of the reported experiences appear not easily explicable in terms solely of similarity judgments. Of course, too, it is obvious that those who notice the redlikeness of a certain sound will be likely also to have called up in their minds an image of red in making the comparison. But this is nothing that anyone might not do, provided he has not so desensualized his imagination as to have become incapable of color images. On the other hand, to observe the redness of a sound the mere word "red" might suffice, as in identifying a red object as such one does not perhaps necessarily recall any previous red experience, or imagine a red additional to that perceived.

In the last few years some rather novel synesthetic doctrines have appeared. An example is R. H. Wheeler's ingenious theory,[58] according to which a per⸺ object, say, to colored hearing is one in whom visual qualities, colors, alone have become developed or actualized, and hence have to take the place of the usual auditory qualities. Such a person "hears as well as anyone else, but he hears visually." He hears colors, whereas others only see them. The presupposition underlying all this seems to be that a thing is either a color or not a color, that the distinction between color qualities and other qualities is absolute and not a matter of degree. If this be so, then I for one am neither synesthetic nor not synesthetic. For I hear (and, like Mr. Wheeler's subject, Mr. Cutsworth, also taste, smell, etc.) qualities something like colors, but seldom if ever exactly like any

[58] See his *Readings in Psychology* (New York, 1930), pp. 358-59.

colors I have seen visually. Sometimes the analogy with color is very clear and fairly closely defined, sometimes it is almost completely elusive, and there are all degrees in between. I see no conclusive evidence that Mr. Cutsworth's experience—or that of a "normal" person—is very different from mine, except that Mr. Cutsworth, having long been blind, has too imperfect a memory of colors to be able to test the accuracy of his color analogies, and the normal person is one who has never become greatly interested in observing intersense likenesses.

When John Burroughs describes the song of the wood thrush as "golden" and two other leading nature writers agree that the (higher-pitched) hermit thrush's song is "silver, burnished silver," are these three persons to be set down as "synesthetic"? Are these descriptions indicative of "photisms" (Wheeler)? If not, what meaning have they? If so, then what person, observant of the subtle nuances of experience, is not a synesthetic subject? Again, since Wheeler asserts that the man who hears colors and only colors nevertheless accurately discriminates all the qualities of sound, e.g., pitch, it is clear that the structure of the color system must be closely parallel to that of the sound system, a fairly strict one-to-one correspondence must obtain. Furthermore, the organismic theory by which Wheeler explains synesthesia is the very one which would favor the abandonment of the doctrine of modes (absolute disparities), and with this abandonment no special explanation would, in most cases at least, be needed, since there would be no phenomenon of synesthesia—except as the observation of likenesses—to explain. In an organism all the parts, being alike organs, display analogies to one another, are more or less akin.

This inference from the organismic conception has, it is a pleasure to discover, recently been drawn. Karl Zietz says:

> All those who speak [in connection with synesthesia] of a subsequent binding together of separate sense impressions, whether directly through associations or in the form of a bridging over [*Überbrückung*], are really adopting the conception of a mosaic-like, agenetic structure of the mental life. The various sensory fields thus appear as disparate systems which constitute starkly isolated "parts" of the mind.
> The place of this "mosaic hypothesis" must however be taken by a "holis-

tic" [*ganzheitliche*] point of view, the life of the mind must be conceived as a living unity. This point of view, which in principle is scarcely opposed to-day, must find concrete application to this special problem of synesthesia.[59]

What are the consequences of this application? By very interesting experimental procedures Zietz shows that color and sound sensations which are simultaneously stimulated not only modify each other, the color altering for instance the pitch of the sound, or the sound the hue of the color, but that the two supposedly heterogeneous sensory elements frequently blend together in experience to such an extent that they are given as one and the same thing. He says:

> Between impressions of tone and of color an objective functional connection is shown to obtain. . . . . Tone and color must, on a deeper level, be something identical.
> In a typical case this functional connection appears also subjectively, as a connection for awareness. Tone and color are then given as identical. [For example, a subject says]: The color itself became the warm, soft tone; [or again:] It [the tone] becomes itself red.[60]

Throughout this monograph results are indicated which correspond to the hypothesis that sound and color are much more alike than different, that indeed a sound may be far more like a certain color than it is like certain other sounds, or than the color is like certain other colors. In short, we have here strong confirmation of the contradictory of Helmholtz' doctrine of modes. These results are not, it is true, "synesthetic." The subjects were normal not synesthetic persons, i.e., not so constituted that stimulation of one sense ordinarily produced automatically imagery belonging to another sense. But Zietz showed that the synesthetic phenomenon could be produced in such subjects as a special case of the experience of intersensory homogeneity, thus verifying the hypothesis that such homogeneity is the objective source and explanation of synesthesia.

What, finally, is the nature, according to Zietz, of the "deeper level" of sensation[61] which constitutes the identity of sound and

---

[59] "Gegenseitige Beeinflussung von Farb- und Tonerlebnissen," *Zeitschrift für Psychologie und Physiologie der Sinnesorgane*, CXXI, 264.

[60] *Ibid.*, pp. 354, 316, 333.

[61] The metaphor of levels is not perhaps very happy—it seems to mean sense data viewed now with regard to those aspects which separate the senses from each other

color? It is that which appears when the sensory processes are seen as "pure bodily-dynamic occurrences." These occurrences, I take it, are feelings, and Zietz quotes Stern to this effect.[62]

The same general approach to synesthesis is found in a number of other German psychologists. The trail, blazed before the dawn of history by the plain man in his "metaphors," i.e., speech comparisons,[63] is now being traveled by the researchers into this much-discussed question.[64]

SECTION 7. THE FAILURE TO PRODUCE AGREEMENT

There is yet a third criterion, besides those of logical structure and relevance to the facts, by which the traditional theory may be tested. We have spoken as though that theory possessed at least the merit of resting upon a great unanimity of opinion. So in fact, in some of its aspects, it does; but the features agreed upon—of what doubtful intrinsic character we have seen—are compensated for, as we shall see in the next two chapters, by the most violent, paradoxical, and seemingly incurable conflicts of opinion. The value of agreement in science lies above all in the means so secured for the attainment of still more extended agreements. Now the tenets concerning sensation held in common by psychological and philosophical schools are, I shall try

---

(e.g., that sounds are less definite in spatial outline) and now with regard to those aspects in which they are one and the same (e.g., in intensity or brightness). The latter is "deeper," for it is the common characters of things in terms of which the most comprehensive laws and, in point of development, the most original causes or sources must be conceived. The peculiar is the superficial, the mere special case.

[62] Stern, *Personalistik als Wissenschaft* (Leipzig, 1930), p. 44.

[63] See von Hornbostel, *Festschrift Meinhof* (1927).

[64] See A. Wellek, "Das Doppelempfinden in der Geistesgeschichte," *Zeitschrift für Aesthetik und allgemeine Kunstwissenschaft*, XXIII, 1; also "Das Doppelempfinden im abendländischen Altertum und Mittelalter," *Archiv für Psychologie*, LXXX, 120; G. Anschütz, "Untersuchungen über complexe musikalische Synopsis," *ibid.*, Vol. LIV; also "Der Farbe-Ton-Problem im psychischen Gesamtbereich," *Deutsche Psychologie*, V, 5; and *Kurze Einführung in die Farbe-Ton Forschung* (Leipzig, 1927); F. Krueger, "Über psychische Ganzheit," *Neue psychologische Studien*, I (1926), 1; Annelies Argeländer, *Das Farbenhören und das synaesthetische Faktor der Wahrnehmung* (Jena, 1927). For a sharp critique of the last-mentioned work see Maria de Bos, *Zeitschrift für Psychologie*, CXI, 321-41, and for a reply to this criticism see G. Anschütz, *ibid.*, CXVI, 309-53. See also Heinz Werner, *Einführung in die Entwicklungspsychologie* (Leipzig, 1926), § 12.

to show, the very ones which are chiefly responsible for their well-known failure to agree upon other fundamental issues, the nature of which is such that direct observation must be capable, if properly applied, of determining the right solutions and of closing the debate. This "proper application" of direct observation is what the traditional theory of sensation effectively discourages. For it holds that there is nothing interesting to observe, nothing scientifically momentous—in a word, no intelligibility—in the qualities of immediate experience. This supposition is not merely unscientific, unfounded; it is also antiscientific—opposed to the spirit of science.

# CHAPTER III

# THE DEADLOCK IN CONTEMPORARY PHILOSOPHY

\*\*

*Those who scorn the certainty of mathematics will find themselves involved in sophistical arguments which end only in a war of words.*

LEONARDO DA VINCI

*The bearing of aesthetics upon abstract intellectual theories has become plain enough. . . . . The questions of epistemology cannot even be formulated without disposing of the given, and the given, provided only that we have an actual meaning for this much-abused word, is the very subject-matter of aesthetic analysis.*

D. W. PRALL

\*\*

### SECTION 8. THE APPEAL TO THE SENSE DATUM

A FAMOUS essay on "The Refutation of Idealism"[1] opens with the following sentences: "Modern idealism, if it asserts any general conclusion about the universe at all, asserts that it is spiritual. There are two points about this assertion to which I wish to call attention. These points are that, whatever be its exact meaning, it is certainly meant to assert (1) that the universe is very different indeed from what it seems, and (2) that it has quite a large number of properties which it does not seem to have. Chairs and tables and mountains seem to be very different from us; but, when the whole universe is declared to be spiritual, it is certainly meant to assert that they are far more like us than we think. The idealist means to assert that they are *in some sense* neither lifeless nor unconscious as they certainly seem to be." Here we have the position that reality, as given concretely or to the senses, is not

---

[1] G. E. Moore, *Mind* (1903) republished in his *Philosophical Studies* (1922), chap. i, with the comment that the author no longer adheres to all of the main features of his earlier view. For the use which I am here making of his essay (to typify a commonly entertained position), Mr. Moore's present adherence to this position is unessential. The quotations from Moore are reprinted by permission of the publishers, Harcourt, Brace and Company, Inc.

in the least mental or spiritual. The remainder of the essay traces this seeming non-spirituality of the universe to that of the sense data which disclose it. The "blue" in the "awareness of blue" does not, Moore says, appear to him as an adjective of the awareness, as though the latter were itself blue, and certainly it cannot be merely such an adjective. Idealism is thus reduced to the conception of sense data as qualities, and not merely objects, of awareness. Is a color, like Boston, in any observable sense, a "state of mind"? Can there be a "blue awareness," Mr. Moore asks?[2]

The same reduction of the issue to a question of observed data is demanded from the idealistic side by Bosanquet. He says:

> The assertion that an object or content has or has not a mental character, ought . . . ., if it has any value, to be supported by *positive analysis, and not merely by extraneous proof. Whether a certain object is continuous with the nature of mind is no question of mere origin or concomitant variation; it is a question of what sort of thing the object is, and what sort of thing the mind is, and whether or no the one is connected with the other by inherent characteristics*. . . . . Now come to a content of sense. What I see when I look at a blue thing has unity and *life*. . . . . It *pulsates with feeling, a common tone,* which involves the presence of a whole all at once, reinforcing and modifying every part by the simultaneous effects of all. What does a unity of this kind consist in? . . . . *Blue is a peculiar "effect," effect, I mean, in the artistic sense* of the word. How do the elements of the effect hold together? What sort of medium does such a unity involve? Surely that of consciousness and no other. . . . . I do not call it "mental" for I am not sure what that means. But I will call it logical.[3]

Again:

> It *seems obvious at first sight that a blue is as psychical as a pain or an inferential transition.* And though you may argue at length that it is nothing but an external object, I feel all the time that I am being defrauded. You have put the vital characteristic of a certain experience into what you call an act, and I admit that it is especially observable in connection with a certain function. But now you tell me that the main thing in the object (what I value in it and what I want it for) is removed and abolished by the distinction, and the experience as such is left for dead. . . . .[4]

[2] Common speech with its "I feel blue" answers this question—with a "metaphor," but nevertheless affirmatively.

[3] B. Bosanquet, *The Distinction between Mind and Its Objects* (Manchester University Press, 1913), pp. 31–33. Reprinted by permission of the publishers. Italics mine.

[4] *Ibid.*, p. 30. Italics mine.

This is surely a flat contradiction, based ostensibly upon observation, of Mr. Moore's position, which also appeals to observation. For Bosanquet psychicality or subjectivity is something positively observable, and observable in the contents of experience, as their constitutive essence. And certainly the supreme misinterpretation of idealism (whether it is the critics of idealism or its defenders that so think) is the notion that its strength consists in maintaining, with Mr. Moore, that consciousness is something *sui generis*, utterly distinct from concrete qualities, inexplicable by them, a mere transparent medium in which the qualities have being.[5] On the contrary, all idealism, even moral, involves seeing at least something akin to the ideal in the simplest and humblest realities, as the basis for the endeavor to embody still more of the ideal in these realities. Idealism means that "the nature of the mind is in everything and the only difficulty is to see it there" (Bosanquet). The key to this perception of the ideal in the real is the notion of value.

> It is a feather in the cap of recent realism to have given the secondary qualities their due. But here its achievements must end. It is impossible on the same principle to do justice to the tertiary qualities, say, beauty or delightfulness. If you reserve aught, for a mind stripped of its objective contents, you must, as realism admits, reserve pleasure and pain..... And whether pain and pleasure are sense-contents or not, I think it has been proved impossible to separate them in treatment from sense-contents..... You must either assign sense-contents to the mind, or aesthetic contents to physical reality.[6]

This is idealism's proper answer to Mr. Moore. Is it a satisfactory one? Bosanquet himself says that he is sure the point could be made much more convincing than he has been able to make it. And the reader may indeed have experienced a certain bewilderment when Bosanquet, after so vividly indicating the emotional character of a color, in the attempt to describe this character further says that, whether or not it is to be termed mental, he will sum up its essence as "logical"! In explanation, however, we learn that the logical is the universal and the universal is of the nature of a conation, a phase of will. All this may be intelligible enough to one well steeped in the idealistic

---

[5] Moore, *Studies*, p. 25.   [6] Bosanquet, *op. cit.*, pp. 36-37.

tradition. But it is not the way to bring about a settlement of the point at issue. The rôle of observation is too subordinated to a somewhat esoteric and partially antiquated terminology. The seemingly implied subordination of feeling to "logic" is precisely the fallacy of explaining the concrete through the abstract upon which, according to idealists, all anti-idealism is based. It is also of a piece with Bosanquet's deterministic monism, his "block universe" in which time is an unintelligible illusion or by-product, in which all that is possible is also actual, an outworn doctrine, as William James so shrewdly saw.

A similar situation confronts us if we survey the idealistic movement in other countries. In Germany, Rickert[7] found himself forced to abandon his master Kant, on the score of "hyletic sensationalism," the doctrine that the entire matter or presented content of external experience consists of mere "sensuous" qualities—that is to say, qualities quite unintelligible to the mind. On the contrary, Rickert holds, the visual or auditory surface of the world is shot through with what he calls intelligible qualities or qualities of value. It is these alone which enable us to attend to objects. If to our ears the wind did not "moan," the thunder "threaten," we should never hear them. In this fashion Rickert's doctrine of truth as a value, earlier presented as a matter of dialectic and of the analysis of the act of belief, is supported by appeal to the data of the senses. Yet this appeal is robbed of most of its effect by the formalistic fashion in which the intelligible qualities are interpreted, namely, as values in the sense of "validities" (*Geltungen*) which are essentially supertemporal in character and the relation of which to the temporal act of sensation can never, Rickert holds, be understood. Thus qualities are not really made intelligible, and we see at once that it is only a kind of transplanted materialism with which we are here confronted. It is precisely matter, as conceived in the nineteenth century, to which the temporal context, like every context, was extrinsic; it is matter which could not be understood in terms of its function in the concrete proc-

[7] Heinrich Rickert, "Die Methode der Philosophie und das Unmittelbare," *Logos*, XII (1923), 235-80.

ess of nature. The old atoms were supertemporal, eternal enough. Rickert's eternal "value forms" are not necessarily an improvement. The old fallacy of merely dissective analysis, responsible for materialism, is repeated here.

One might go on to mention many thinkers of note (e.g., Heidegger) who hold the same view but who fail in one way or another to present the issue in a trenchant fashion, couched in terms of the modes of thinking which science and practical life have made dominant in our era. The realists have appeared to be talking the language of common-sense and scientific sobriety, the idealists that of lofty special insight or baseless fancies. They have even gloried, sometimes, in this aristocratic aloofness. They have had their reward! Who has understood Croce's intention in his "identification" of intuition and expression? Apparently, of those not already of a similar way of thinking, scarcely anyone, outside of Italy at least.[8]

The general upshot is that many opponents of idealism do not seem even to know that such an idealistic appeal to the datum has been made, although almost every idealist in history has in fact made it. Thus the two groups of thinkers have failed to join issue upon the observational problem. This failure can be exemplified in the very founder of modern idealism. The remarks of Berkeley to which I refer have passed, so far as I have been able to ascertain, substantially without notice. This is partly, no doubt, in consequence of the somewhat casual fashion in which they occur in the course of Berkeley's dialectical argument; but even more, assuredly, to the unreadiness of the modern mind to take seriously the order of facts to which Berkeley has reference. If proof of the strength of this prejudice were needed, we could find it here. But even Berkeley himself seems to treat the phenomena in question merely as furnishing one among many of the links in the chain of his argument for idealism. Like other modern thinkers, he had turned to sensations,

---

[8] See Croce's article on "Aesthetics" in the *Encyclopaedia Britannica* (14th ed.) for perhaps the clearest account of the doctrine. Leo Stein, in his *A B C of Aesthetics*, and Lascelles Abercrombie, in his *Towards a Theory of Art*, are among the few whose references to Croce indicate understanding of, in spite of a decidedly critical attitude toward, his doctrines.

not to find out what they were like, but to collect evidence for the truth or falsity of a philosophical theory whose main interest and bearings lay elsewhere. Nevertheless, Berkeley possessed enough psychological curiosity and acuteness to make, as is well known, some notable discoveries in the field of sensory phenomena. A good example is his series of observations bearing upon the relation of certain of our external sensations to the feelings of pleasure and pain.

"Is not the most vehement and intense degree of heat a very great pain? .... And is any unperceiving thing capable of pain or pleasure?" (Hylas, at first, concedes the point, but then, in order to escape the idealistic inference, revises his position: "I fear I was out in yielding intense heat to be a pain. It should seem rather, that pain is something distinct from heat, and the consequence or effect of it." Philonus replies:)

"Upon putting your hand near the fire, do you perceive one simple uniform sensation, or two distinct sensations?"

"But one simple sensation."

"Is not the heat immediately perceived?"

"It is."

"And the pain?"

"True."

"Seeing therefore they are both immediately perceived at the same time, and the fire affects you only with one simple or uncompounded idea, it follows that this simple idea is both the intense heat immediately perceived, and the pain, and consequently that the intense heat immediately perceived is nothing distinct from a particular sort of pain?"

"It seems so."

"Again, try in your thoughts, Hylas, if you can conceive a vehement sensation to be without pain or pleasure? .... Or can you frame to yourself an idea of sensible pain or pleasure in general in abstraction from every particular idea of heat, cold, tastes, smells? etc."

"I do not find that I can."

"Doth it not therefore follow, that sensible pain is nothing distinct from those sensations or ideas, in an intense degree? .... And is not warmth, or a more gentle degree of heat than what causes uneasiness, a pleasure? .... If you are resolved to maintain that warmth, or a gentle degree of heat, is not pleasure, I know not how to convince you otherwise than by appealing to your own sense." (The argument is then applied to cold, which "in intense degree" at least is admitted to be a pain. The case of mild coldness leads aside to a very different line of argument. We then return to the affective interpretation as follows:)

"Is a sweet taste a particular kind of pleasure or pleasant sensation, or is it not? .... Is not bitterness some kind of uneasiness or pain? .... In the next place *odours*, .... are they not so many pleasing or displeasing sensations?"[9]

[9] Berkeley, *First Dialogue between Hylas and Philonus.*

Although the specific examples which Berkeley gives are those of heat, taste, and odors, the fully generalized arguments quoted above concerning the identity of pains or pleasures, ordinarily so called, with intense sensations, together with the express denial in the *Commonplace Book* that any sensations can be entirely "indifferent" or without intrinsic relation to the will,[10] reveal that Berkeley's idealism involved the thesis that as a matter of observational fact the intuited contents ordinarily known as affective, and almost universally admitted to belong exclusively to the mind, do not represent a special genus or unique principle in contrast to the supposed mere or neutral contents, but rather, as Leibniz had said, the "most notable" or unmistakable examples[11] of a principle of value which careful introspection reveals as constitutive of all experience.

On the other hand, it would be far too much to claim that Berkeley took full advantage of his opportunities. The difficulties of his system: the heterogeneity of contents of awareness and awareness itself, consequently of the "ideas" and "notions" by which respectively the two were known; the lack—exploited by Hume with such deadly effect—of organic relation among ideas, and the ghostlike or shadow reality of a world composed of wholly "inert" ideas or percepts—so rightly found unconvincing on sound empirical evidence by Dr. Johnson—all these and other well-known difficulties were in principle overcome by the affective interpretation of sensation. At least, they would have been so if the distinction between self-feelings and object-feelings, and the resultant social conception of perception as a transaction with finite entities real on the same plane as ourselves (although, as Leibniz held, akin to us, spiritual not dead or material), had been recognized and developed. But it is only too clear that in the face of many of these difficulties it did not occur to Berkeley to employ his affective principle to solve them. The influence of the intellectualism, the very materialism even, of his age was far too strong. Berkeley's "ideas" were for

[10] Fraser's ed., p. 53.
[11] See also Berkeley, *Commonplace Book*, ed. Fraser, pp. 39 and 62.

many purposes only dead material objects transplanted into mind.

The assumption against which Berkeley should have directed a far more explicit attack is beautifully expressed by John Locke:

> Amongst the simple ideas which we receive both from sensation and reflection, pain and pleasure are two very considerable ones. For as in the body there is sensation barely in itself, or accompanied with pain or pleasure; so the thought or perception of the mind is simply so, or else accompanied also with pleasure or pain, delight or trouble, call it how you please. . . . . . Things then are good or evil only in reference to pleasure or pain.[12]

This idea that there may be sensations, perceptions, which are "simply so," this idea of "bare" awareness has been representative almost throughout the modern era.[13] The fact par excellence is what is "simply so"; it is an addition to the bare fact if it has relation to value. That bareness with respect to value turns out to be bareness with respect to intelligibility also, that a fact which was simply "so" would be simply nothing for attention and interest, or that enjoyment is not the "accompaniment" of life, but life itself—all this is naïvely overlooked. Elsewhere Locke says that ideas of pleasure and pain are "annexed" to our other ideas. We might call this the annex view of value. But according to idealism it is the living mind that dwells in this annex, while in the supposed main building are nothing but the haunting ghosts of abstractionist mythologies, of materialistic verbalisms.

To Locke's conception of the possible neutrality of sensations, Leibniz, that profound idealist before Berkeley, could not agree. He says: "I believe that there are no perceptions which are wholly indifferent to us, but it is enough that their effect be not notable in order that they may be thus spoken of, for *pleasure* and *pain* appear to consist in a notable aid or impediment."[14] This is an excellent example of the way in which his principle

---

[12] *Essay*, Book II, chap. xx, § 1.

[13] See A. N. Whitehead's presidential address, "Objects and Subjects," *Philosophical Review*, XLI, No. 3 (1932), 130 ff.; also in *Proceedings of the American Philosophical Association*, Vol. V; and in *Adventures of Ideas*, chap. xi.

[14] *New Essays*, trans. Langley (1916), Book II, chap. xx, p. 167.

of continuity enabled Leibniz to transcend the rough discriminations of common sense. In everyday life what are called pleasures and pains are the most intense phases of the affective life; the rest, being of importance only as clues to the environment, are classified as "non-affective." This means that their value as use far outweighs their value as enjoyment. Only one who by mathematical training had learned that a great and for ordinary purposes complete difference may still be but a matter of degree, that a character may be ever so small and still not sink to absolute zero—or else one accustomed to discriminate experience for the direct enjoyment of its finer flavors—would be likely to see the relativity of the sensation-affection distinction. Leibniz doubtless came to the matter chiefly from the mathematical standpoint.

Thus we might go on to show how such representative idealists as Plato, Hegel, Schelling, Schopenhauer—in fact, almost all idealists, unless Kant be an exception—have recognized in the directly perceived character of the datum as such a part of the evidence for the spiritual interpretation of reality. This perceived character, implicative of spiritualism, has been the aesthetic or emotional content of the given. No idealist, unless Kant be one, has ever committed himself to the generic separation of sense data from values; all have pointed to facts which negate this distinction. On the other hand, this phase of the evidence has not, until recent times, been made as central to the argument as the hard-won modern conviction of the importance of verifying generalities through concrete and particular perceptions implies that it should be. In view of the slowness with which the human mind has learned—is still learning—the complete necessity for this factual verification, there is nothing surprising in the historic emphasis upon argument at the expense of specific publicly verifiable perceptions.

### SECTION 9. THE STATUS OF TERTIARY QUALITIES

If the basis of idealism is the essentially aesthetic quality of sense data, then the criticism of idealism may take one of two forms. It may be said, and has been said, that aesthetic or tertiary characters are indeed given as belonging to sense objects, but as not necessarily involving anything so psychological as "feeling." The object, apart from mind and feeling, may be beautiful, ugly, or the like. The admitted consequence is to make such predicates inexplicable. Moreover, so far this position has proved hopelessly incredible to most persons. Finally, it does not meet the contention of idealists that not merely aesthetic values, but specifically these values as feelings, are given as objective contents in sensation.

The second alternative open to idealism's critics is to deny the intrinsically aesthetic character of sense data. This denial has frequently been made. Professor Perry, for instance, finds no trace of aesthetic qualities in extrabodily phenomenal space.[15] Thus upon the very threshold of perception the old conflict of opinions emerges, apparently as insoluble as it is in its dialectical formulation. Must the cause of agreement be given up and temperament, prejudice, or differing degrees of "insight" be admitted the determining factors? I for one cannot accept this conclusion, cannot believe that so clear an issue, appealing so directly to the simplest and commonest of perceptual experiences, can forever remain at the mercy of desires and beliefs which have no clear justification at their command. If the realist sees nothing of an aesthetic or affective character in external experience, while the idealist sees nothing else, and if both really mean "see" and not rather believe or know, then the difficulty cannot lie essentially either in personal idiosyncrasies of a sensuous character or in mere differences of abstract belief or general philosophical preferences, nor in a combination of all these. For the conflict of opinions is more radical than all such differences put together. If we take the idealist and the realist each at his word, the implication is that between the two proposed pictures of sense experience there is nothing in common: whatever one may be, the other is through and through and utterly not that! This is not a difference such as that between a sensitive and an insensitive person, or between an imaginative, speculative, and

[15] See R. B. Perry, *Journal of Philosophy*, March, 1914, p. 153; or his *General Theory of Value* (New York, 1926), pp. 31 ff., 284-91.

a sober, matter-of-fact, type of mind, or between the religious and the irreligious. For all such differences are relative only, whereas this appears to be absolute.

Surely the best conclusion from the resulting impasse is that neither of the two parties has succeeded in conveying to the other what the question at issue is conceived to be, so that each in resorting to observation is testing a different hypothesis from the other. They do not see the same things, because, perhaps, they are not looking for the same things. That they do not discover this must be due to some mistaken premiss concerning the manner in which the terms used are to be defined; and the failure to correct this premiss arises, in turn, in all probability, from its not having been brought to full consciousness by either party. It is because some of men's agreements are mistaken that so many of their disagreements seem incurable. It is what we concede to one another that keeps us apart!

Now in fact such a mistaken common assumption is involved in the very term "tertiary quality." This term suggests that in the external sensory realm there are, so to say, layers of properties, one upon the other, so that in tabulating the contents of that realm one admits first of all such entities as colors, sounds, and the like, and then as an addition, such a character as, say, the "sweetness" of such-and-such a sound. The very admission of "tertiary" characters appears historically as an afterthought. The term itself is ambiguous; it means (*a*) characters of an aesthetic, emotional, or evaluational character, or (*b*) simply whatever is still left in sensory experience when we abstract the primary and secondary characters, the space-time configurations, the colors, and sounds, etc. Now these two meanings ought to be sharply distinguished and the status of each discussed separately. The position of idealism amounts to the doctrine that, just as shapes, sizes, motions, and the like are nothing without some sort of secondary qualities to form the content of these more abstract forms, so, and in a still more absolute sense, secondary qualities are nothing without the aesthetic feelings to which they are merely a formalized reference. But this radical reversal of history, making the last first, has been too profound a breaking with tradition for even its own prophets to see it altogether clearly and consistently. The absolute centrality of value, which is the gist of idealism, has not been given a clear technical expression, either in general or in this specific instance. It has not been consistently and emphatically proclaimed, else it would have been more commonly seen, that a character may be aesthetic without for all that falling outside the class of primary and secondary qualities, i.e., without being more or other than just a shape or a color or a smell or a taste! Thus the term "tertiary" does not necessarily stand for the addition of a new species of quality, but rather for the addition of a new interpretation of the species already recognized though not yet properly understood. The feeling tone of a color is not, according to an idealism that understands itself, something over and above the color; it is just the color itself seen in its intelligible essence. The "mere" color again is not something less or more than its aesthetic content; it is simply an impoverished, more purely denotative mode of reference to that same content. It is a difference of adequacy of concepts, not a difference of objects referred to.

In contrast to all this, most critics of idealism, in looking for tertiary qualities without the organisms, have obviously supposed the goal of their search to be entities distinct from the mere sensory qualities of color and the like. Actual scrutiny, on the contrary, reveals to them that the only qualities in aesthetic experience which are anything more than just the sensations themselves are feelings within the body, reverberations of the bodily "sounding board." Here the idealist may well agree. Indeed, as will be shown later (sec. 13), sensory determinations exhaust the qualitative potentialities of the portions of phenomenal space which they occupy.

On the other hand, when the critic of idealism denies the occurrence of tertiary qualities in extrabodily phenomenal space, he comes into conflict with facts. The most careful experimental work that has been done in several countries to determine this very question has clearly established the contrary position. "Objective feelings" are observed facts. The opponent of idealism must adopt an interpretation of these facts which, whether true or false, is certainly debatable. And the point is, it is not being debated, except indirectly and hastily, by philosophers whose difference of philosophic standpoint implies opposite decisions in regard to it. For this failure to debate the crucial point neither party to the controversy can be held solely responsible.

### SECTION 10. QUALITY AND INTEREST

The more or less unconscious disagreement concerning objective feelings to which we have traced the philosophical impasse is correlated with a similar possible disagreement concerning subjective feelings. The most definitive exposition of the anti-idealistic view is again furnished by Professor Perry in his much-discussed theory of value. The crux of this theory for our purposes is the definition which it proposes of affection, i.e., pleasantness-unpleasantness. This definition posits two ingredients: somatic sensation and the attitude of interest having such sensation as its objects. The relation to interest is held to be extrinsic to the quality of the sensation, but is by definition intrinsic to "affection"; that is to say, affection is somatic sensation which, as a sheer addition to its sensory character, arouses interest.[16] The latter is a bodily response, and both it and its objects are describable in terms of neutral entities not involving mind or interest in their natures. The logic of absolute atomistic analysis reaches here one of its most perfect expressions.

One implication of this view is that it is quite possible to conceive a being to whom keen pain, bitter tastes, and the odor of sulphur would be intensely delectable, while the qualities of sex sensations, sweet tastes, flowery odors, as we now have them, would be no less intensely distasteful and repellant. Now it is true that the variations in men's tastes might plausibly be used as evidence of this possibility, subject, however, to critical considerations earlier brought forward, and in opposition to the extraordinarily pertinacious conviction upon which hedon-

---

[16] A similar view is expressed by Dickinson S. Miller, "The Pleasure-Quality and the Pain-Quality Analyzable, Not Ultimate," *Mind*, N.S., XXXVIII, 215-18.

ism in all forms is based that pleasure represents both quality and psychic acceptance in a real fusion, not in a compound of two externally related factors. The main trend of psychological opinion seems also always to have favored a qualitative view of acceptance-rejection.

It is not, however, necessary to rely on such convictions. There are also matters of logical principle involved. One of these three things must be true: mind is an organic whole; it is just what the American New Realists say it is, a pattern of externally related simples; or it is a sheer mystery, as Mr. G. E. Moore seems to hold. The last view offers nothing to science, which is not acquainted with any criteria of inexplicability. The second view is open to the same objection, since its simples are nothing but such illegitimate inexplicables. The first view, which is idealism, implies not that the object of human knowing is merely a state of that knowing, but that when the object is humanly known it becomes also such a state, whatever other status it may have. The given expresses the intuition to or for or by which it is given. The question, however, then becomes: How does red, say, involve the context of experience in which it occurs? The only clear answer seems to me to be in terms of just such an intrinsic relation as one seems to intuit between the quality of pleasure and the function of interest, and such further relations of interfusion as are grounded upon this, or are similar to it.

An objection to the doctrine of mind as a congeries of simples is that it destroys the meaning of the idea of individuality. Simples have nothing to prevent their repetition in various contexts, hence they are universals. Complexes, externally derived from these universals, are only complex universals, and it is rather too much to ask us to believe that this is all there is to the age-old problem of the *principium individuationis*. The fact is that individuality is identifiable only by direct grasp of a thing as a "this," that is to say through its relations to the experiential context. The individual and real is what acts upon and is acted upon by us. The relative or approximate independence of the real object from ourselves as subject is the protean and social character of the latter, its lack of absolute severance from other actual and possible selves. There is for idealism, or at least for spiritualism, no self except that which is a member of all other selves and of which they are members. He who thinks that the world, without any such unity of significance as constitutes an experience, would still have been or might be a real world, and who deduces this from the fact—which spiritualism accepts—that the world without a particular human personality, Mr. X, is perfectly possible, must also be one who thinks that if from "himself" those qualities and relations which make him Mr. X were to be subtracted, nothing of the nature of mind would remain—in short, he is one who does not believe that other minds are members of himself. Such sheer privacy is the essence of what I call "materialism." For the contrary or spiritualistic doctrine, Mr. X is a social organism seen in a unique perspective in one of its members.[17] Imagine the suppression of that member and you do not imagine the complete destruction of the organism but only its more or less slight or profound alteration, according to the importance of the member in question. The self imagining itself to vanish, in another sense imagines itself to remain, namely, the sense in which it already identifies itself with other selves, actual and possible, human and non-human, the sense in which it overlaps and is one with them.

Idealism is absolute spiritualism, or it is a miserable compromise which history has already condemned. Its triumph would mean that we really believed that we are our neighbors—individuated from them none the less by the Leibnizian-Whiteheadian principle of relative degrees of vividness in the sensing of the qualities of existence. Such belief can only come as all culture advances, including ethical—so that we no longer give it the lie by preaching or accepting self-interest as the sole efficacious motive of conduct. The whole economic structure of society might have to be altered in this process. Meanwhile it is incumbent upon both protagonists and critics of the spiritualist

---

[17] See Whitehead's analysis in *Adventures of Ideas*, chaps. xi-xiii, or in *Process and Reality*, Part III.

doctrine to try to clear the issue of inconsistent combinations of the only two possible doctrines: (1) matter, that which is not one with us through immediate sociality, sympathetic *rapport*, does or at least may possibly exist; (2) no such matter can exist. The former doctrine is no more "realistic" than the latter; for the social relation has a term as real as the subject of the relation, and if this relation is categorically essential—as spiritualism holds—then its term must include something immediately given, embraced in the subject. Among the half-hearted idealisms none are more lukewarm, it seems to me, than those which accept a quasi-solipsistic exclusion of all neighbors from immediacy. The whole question just is whether immediacy is or is not social in essence.

Value is clearly the object of interest, but according to idealism only because interest is itself an object of interest and indeed the only interesting thing; because interest and value are one in socialized affection, the primordial material of life out of which analysis produces, by selective emphasis, such relatively diverse concepts as interest and sense quality.

The question returns upon us: Is this doctrine observationally true? It is time, in seeking to answer this question, to consider the qualifications of philosophers as observers of immediacy.

### SECTION 11. THE PHILOSOPHER AS OBSERVER

Philosophers are eager to distinguish their "acquaintance" with sense data from their "knowledge about" them. But philosophers are not altogether fitted by mental habits and interests to succeed in this. They are much more sincerely interested in concepts and knowledge about than in sheer data. They are in fact interested in the latter not for their own sakes but almost solely as starting-points of more knowledge about. "What other interest could there be?" you may ask. I answer, "A genuine interest not indeed solely in the data in themselves, exclusively for their own sakes, but at least partially so." And this interest, in so far as it is interest in knowledge about, should be in knowledge relevant to what the things are in themselves. Now if one has been taught to think that things are ineffable, then one will suppose that no knowledge about can be verified by what the things are intuited to be in themselves. Thus the doctrine of absolute simplicity or unintelligibility precludes any cognitive interest in the data themselves and limits this interest to the discernment of relations which need have been no different had the qualities in themselves been other than they are. But further, interest in knowledge about even of a sort germane to the data in themselves pre-supposes another and non-conceptual interest, a purely intuitional interest, a delight in seeing the thing, or, more accurately, since the attention must be on the object, a delight in the thing as seen. What is this interest, not in knowing, but first of all just in having the datum? Surely, this is no recondite mystery. The delight of beholding just to behold is the aesthetic delight. The only object which can be vividly known by acquaintance is the aesthetic object. But philosophers have been taught that their task is first of all to see things not for their values but for their mere "factual" qualities, i.e., not aesthetically.

I conclude from these considerations that philosophers have been trebly barred from success in their attempt to study the sense data, for (1) they have mainly wanted to know something else (the truth about idealism and the like); (2) they have believed there was nothing to know but only something to intuit; (3) they have believed that the only psychologically possible mode of intuition was not relevant. The result has been that the actual nature of sense experience has been less fully grasped by philosophers than by many other classes of men.

An "idealist" we may now describe as a philosopher who is at least partially free from the foregoing three disqualifications for sensory study. He has had a little more curiosity about the data themselves (evidence, *inter alia*, Hegel's and Schopenhauer's interest in Goethe's color theory); his doctrine at least suggests that sense qualities, being manifestations of mind, should be intelligible to mind; and idealists have at least never been so sure as their critics of the irrelevance of aesthetic intuition.

If it is asked what classes of persons should be least hampered by the prejudices in question, we can hardly be in doubt of the answer. Recollections from early childhood make it clear that the sensory surfaces of things then held one's fascinated attention. There are similar reasons for turning to the racial childhood, to primitive man, whose interest in his immediately given environment was less conceptualized, more unrestrictedly absorbed, in moments of no practical urgency, in merely experiencing the world about him. Thus it is not surprising that Ernst Cassirer in studying the origins of symbolism should have intensified his idealistic impression of the quality of immediate objects. His conclusion is that awareness is more rather than less directly social awareness of other mind and of meaning than it is awareness of mere things or non-mental qualities. He states this as the datum "invariably" gained by "sinking ourselves in pure perception."[18] He also points out that unless the world had "seemed" to the savage the sort of thing his mythologies pictured it to be, these mythologies would have seemed nonsense to him—indeed, could never have been thought of. This mythological world, which was also the apparent world of perception, involved two main characteristics—it involved a social relation of subject and object and it involved continuity of qualities and kinds of things. As to the one, Cassirer says:

> From the purely genetic standpoint, also, there seems to be no doubt which of the two forms of perception is to be regarded as prior. The farther back we trace perception the more in it the form of the "You" gains over the form of the "It," the more clearly the character of expression dominates over that of fact and thing. The "understanding of expression" is essentially earlier than the "knowing of things."[19] [As to the other point, we read:] The myth shows us a world which is not indeed by any means without structure, without immanent differentiation, but which is yet lacking in differentiation according to real "things" and "properties." On the contrary the forms of existence show here a peculiar "fluidity"; .... each of them is to a certain extent ready at any moment to change itself into another of seemingly quite opposite character..... For them there are no logical kinds .... on the contrary all boundary lines drawn by our empirical concepts of genera and species are here evaded.....[20]

[18] Ernst Cassirer, *Philosophie der symbolischen Formen*, III, 73–78.

[19] *Ibid.*, p. 74. See also Heinz Werner, *Einführung in die Entwicklungspsychologie* (Leipzig, 1926), §§ 10 and 35.

[20] *Op. cit.*, pp. 71–72.

## § 11  DEADLOCK IN CONTEMPORARY PHILOSOPHY

Unless, Cassirer remarks, direct experience itself exhibited some real continuity of this sort, the myth would have "hung in a vacuum," and have represented a purely pathological exception instead of a universal human phenomenon.

From the racial childhood let us turn to the civilized child. In his well-known works Jean Piaget[21] shows that it is only with the greatest difficulty that the child learns to see in the external world any different sort of reality from what he feels himself to be. This is partly because motion is to the child, as an observer of animals can hardly doubt it is to animals, simply the manifest presence of life. This experience is a feeling before it is a thought; as immediately given, motion is an aliveness. Moreover, there is at first no sharp sense of distinction between the life within and the life without. Something like the complete reverse of the conception of datum and awareness as totally heterogeneous is, for many years, the only idea the child has. "Continuity" is the basic form of his apprehensions.

Of course we will be told that the child cannot analyze or discriminate. But the child certainly does make plenty of discriminations. Things are not "all alike" to him by any means. What is true is that the supposed dichotomy of emotional and material or neutral entities is to the child practically imperceptible. It would be a strange explanation of the inability of untutored experience to see that two things both immediately given are greatly different, to suppose that the two in fact as immediately given are devoid of similarity. The analogy of the child's own body to moving objects is irrelevant to the main problem— which is why there is not a sharp sense of the difference between this very body, as given by secondary quality intuitions, and the self as given in emotions of longing, fear, etc.

Piaget unfortunately fails to question the children concerning secondary qualities as such; in fact, he shows a slightly amusing inability vividly to appreciate the child's point of view. He has evidently almost forgotten his own childhood. It is also interesting to the idealist to note that the reasons which lead the child to abandon panpsychism as he grows older are totally ir-

---

[21] I have in mind chiefly his *Child's Conception of the World* (New York, 1929), esp. pp. 130, 227-37.

relevant to the logic of the case. These reasons, apart from the authority of elders, are all equivalent to this: that the detailed predictions of behavior which the child deduces from its notions of the wills in things prove mistaken. Logically this proves only that his detailed conceptions of these wills are erroneous. It proves nothing about the principle of panpsychism except that the experiences of ordinary life, plus some smatterings of science, do not suffice to give determinate application of this principle to particular events. But as far back as Leibniz panpsychism accepted physics, and not naïve experience, as its authority in matters of detail.

At any rate, the evidence is that, by any ordinary meaning of the word, the world "seems," at least to the savage, to children, and to certain highly cultivated and intellectual persons, a realm of feeling in continuity with feeling—in short, spiritual. Anti-idealism as an appeal to publicly observable facts has failed to make out its case. So, if you will, has idealism. There is need for an improved technique of observation and analysis in order that we may distinguish between really seeming and merely seeming to seem—in short, between sound and unsound observations of immediate phenomena.

In attempting to devise such a technique, philosophers should not overlook the existence of an experimental science which appears to be concerned with the very same problem—the science of introspective psychology. It is curious how blankly unaware many philosophical disputants appear to be of the data and methods which psychologists have recently arrived at in their inquiry into the epistemologically central question of the nature of sensory experience. Any comparable ignoring of the results of physics or biology would be considered absurd. Problematic as the scientific status of introspective psychology may be, such a degree of unsophistication concerning its results is hardly becoming to any philosopher who aspires to a solution of the epistemological problem.[22]

[22] The relevance of psychological data to this problem has been affirmed by one psychologist at least, who reads them as establishing the truth of idealism—not, however, the realistic or social idealism defended in this book. See C. Spearman, *The Nature of Intelligence* (London, 1923), chap. xiv, and pp. 241-50, 354; also Spearman, *Creative Mind* (London and Cambridge, 1930), chap. xi.

## CHAPTER IV

## THE CONFLICT OF OPINIONS IN PSYCHOLOGY
**\*\***

*I should insist that psychology begin with the life-impulse as its datum, and that it be concerned with the mental routes by which the impulse expresses itself.*

L. L. THURSTONE

*The sensory qualities are also, and demonstrably, spiritual qualities.*

EDOUARD SPRANGER

**\*\***

### SECTION 12. SENSATION AND FEELING

IN THE preceding chapter it was shown that the current theory of sensation, in its philosophical form, lacks even the merit of eliciting unanimous acceptance, and that the disagreements to which it has increasingly led are such as to offer little hope of remedy except through the definite abandonment of the theory. We have now to ask whether a similar case can be made out in psychology. To what extent is sensory materialism, as defined in section 3 and criticized in chapter ii, productive of mutual understanding and reasonable unanimity of opinion among experimental psychologists? Are any of the latter irreconcilable opponents of the "prevailing" doctrine, and how strong is their position?

In considering this question we must remember that the alternative to materialism in sensory theory is a view which integrates sensations and affections into a single system with common dimensional characters which are more naturally suggested by the term "feeling" than by the term "sensation." Now the basic conflict of doctrines in psychology does not obviously turn upon the question of the relation between sense and feeling. This conflict, which is of course that between introspective and behavioristic tendencies, shows, however, such striking analogy to the philosophical deadlock of idealism and realism that we cannot but surmise that the dependence of the latter dispute upon the sensory question will have its counterpart in the psychological controversy. That this is, in fact, the case is the conclusion to which the present chapter tends. Either introspectionism must be given up, or sensory materialism must be discredited. Behaviorism, in the sense of the reduction of mind to matter, has as its overt or covert premiss a false report upon the nature of sensory phenomena as directly observable. And its falsity is beginning to be recognized, as introspective methods are refined and rendered more exact. The future of introspectionism is bound up, it begins to appear, with the future of the affective continuum.

In general, psychology is, in its present state, decidedly more favorable to the doctrine of the affectivity of sensations than it has ever been before. All the great advances in recent times encourage the conviction that the idea of neutral, non-appreciative awareness—"bare awareness," it might be called—is a self-contradictory abstraction; that apart from factors of motive and valuation, apart from aesthetic and emotional aspects, nothing recognizable remains of consciousness or experience. All the great shifts of emphasis—from contents or elements to functional drives, from atomic parts to organic wholes, from conscious "idea" to subconscious "wish," from the private to the social, from the having of data to the reacting with and adjustment to the environment, nay even the behaviorist's attempted substitution of the organism, the strongest reactions of which are the emotional, for "consciousness" — all are forces in this direction. Yet, on the whole, opinions stand against a too close assimilation of sensation and affection; and, although a few highly general and indefinite suggestions pointing in this direction have been made, it scarcely seems that psychology is yet ready to attempt to explain sensation through its analogies with affectivity. The most that can be said is that the older attempt to explain affectivity through sensation is not in much favor.[1] But that it is the business of science to exhaust the possibilities of explanation of the apparently inexplicable elements confronting

[1] But see sec. 15 for a discussion of an important renewal of this attempt.

it, and that therefore if sensation does not explain affection it is the duty of psychology to attempt, in the most resolute way, to explain sensation through affectivity, this, it seems, has occurred to few. He who denies this duty should explain how, if scientists of the past had thus been willing to accept apparent barriers to explanation as real ones, science could have progressed!

The need of an affective explanation of sensation appears further from the account of the self which is in general favor in contemporary psychology. The challenge of Hume to furnish an observable reality for the idea of "self" or of consciousness as distinct from its imaginal "contents" has been met by psychology with unwonted agreement chiefly in one way, the description of the self, or of the mind, in terms of the organic continuity or interfusion of the so-called elements of which the mind is conscious of being composed. The term "soul" turns out to stand for the fact that a mind is all of one piece, that it has aspects rather than self-sufficient atom-like parts. Above all, the self, the person, stands for the unity of the stream of consciousness through time; and this unity is mediated not only by conscious memory as well as by the time breadth of the specious present, but also and fundamentally by the persistence of more or less unconscious desires and emotional attitudes, together with the more conscious moods and purposes. If this doctrine (and psychology seems to have no other except the return to an unexplained unobservable "soul," on the one hand, and sheer materialistic behaviorism, on the other) is really to be taken seriously—and I, for one, believe it is one of the greatest of all scientific discoveries—then I submit that it implies that consciousness or mind as such is an emotional and purposive organism, with the obvious corollary that nothing can enter into the consciousness of a person except as it fulfils or positively frustrates those desires or purposes which constitute his personality; in short, except as values, positive or negative. If, therefore, one distinguishes two aspects of contents, the qualitative and the affective, the former will then not really be included in the unity of the conscious self as defined, and we shall find ourselves thrown back upon Mc-

Dougall's "soul," a word for the problem, nothing more, or upon vague metaphors like the "stream of consciousness"—in short, substantially upon the Humian problem (or else upon dogmatic denials of mind as anything more than physical motions of the body).[2] There is no scientific value in ascribing organization to conscious contents unless we can observe something of the principles, the basic hows of this "interpenetration"; but, as the best glimpses we can get of such unity, taken from the most central standpoints, are all glimpses into the persistence and controlling power of the wish or the purpose or the affective tone, it seems simply reckless neglect of the clues proffered us for the interpretation of more peripheral, less influential aspects, such as sensation, to conclude too lightly from more or less biased observations that sensations cannot be explained upon an affective basis.

In more behavioristic terms the argument can be stated as follows. The nervous system seems to have two main functions: one is to induce action on the part of the organism; the other is passively to receive impressions of the state of affairs within and without the organism. Yet the integral character of the nervous arc warns us not to exaggerate the distinction. Moreover, the state of affairs within the organism includes dispositions to act, and an inseparable aspect of such dispositions as conscious seems to be feeling, so that the receiving of impressions and the initiating of actions seem to become one in this phenomenon. Also, passivity is only the partial dependence of one activity upon another, so that if we are conscious of ourselves as passive we are conscious of the environment as active. If, then, the form in which active tendencies become conscious is feeling, it appears that we must be aware of the environment as itself having feelings. Certainly from the logical standpoint it cannot be denied

[2] How elusive consciousness, so treated, may become is well shown in the following passage from an English philosopher (G. E. Moore, *Studies*, p. 25): ". . . . The moment we try to fix our attention upon consciousness to see *what*, distinctly, it is, it seems to vanish: it seems as if we had before us a mere emptiness. When we try to introspect the sensation of blue, all we can see is the blue: the other element is as it were diaphanous. Yet it *can* be distinguished if we look attentively enough, and if we know that there is something to look for."

that the difference between reception and reaction posited by the reflex act might be fully covered in conscious terms by the distinction between feelings received as (1) those (either illusorily or actually) belonging to the environment and (2) those felt as constituting part and parcel of that dominating core of experience which is "one's self." And finally we have to remember that "of the two functions that have been attributed to receptors, the capacity to excite action and the ability to initiate impulses for sensation, the former is much the more widely distributed of the two and is without question the more primitive."[3] There are animals whose sense receptors are not connected with any central nervous pathways such as are involved in sense perception; and the differentiation of nervous tissue is preceded—and seems, as it were, elicited—by the differentiation of muscle tissue. Thus the primitive function of the senses is action and not information. How strange, then, to regard the feeling tone which is admittedly a normal factor in sense experience, and is the only intrinsic reference to action which the experience as conscious involves, as though it were a mere associative accretion, instead of, as the biological data indicate, the primordial matrix out of which sensory qualities are evolved, the very stuff out of which they are made! The first layer of sensory awareness must be the sense of activity, and the subsequent associative addition can only be the objectification of this activity feeling upon the environment, together with the intellectualization of the direct feeling content, that is, its entanglement in a web of interconnections which tend to weaken the interest in its actual intrinsic (emotional) character. It is not the objectified feeling tone which is an illusory addition to the hard fact of the sensory quality, but rather it is the notion of a mere neutral action-indifferent quality which is an introspective illusion, wholly associative in origin. Upon this illusion psychologies as well as philosophies have been, and are still being, founded.

The matter may be put still otherwise. Feeling is the sense of what the animal inclines to do. But the animal needs also a

[3] G. H. Parker, *Smell, Taste, and Allied Senses in the Vertebrates* (1922), p. 21.

sense of what the environment may be expected to do. Now in what terms shall the animal sense the active tendencies of the environment? It cannot form an abstract concept of "energy" in the lifeless sense of physics. There is only one thing it can do, namely, feel the (real or illusory) feelings and desires of the environment. If primitive man was unable to conceive the physical in abstraction from the psychical, in particular from volitions and emotions, how much less must animals be capable of escaping this panpsychic form of apprehension! And what is each of us in so far as our sensations and affections alone are considered but an animal? This is in addition to the fact that the most important features of the animal's environment are unquestionably those which concern the activities of other animals. An inevitable question, therefore, is whether sensation is essentially the meeting-point of self with "things"—as pure "not-selves"—or of self with self in the form of social fellow. And, be it not forgotten, the most immediate contact of sensation, as nearly all admit, is with what are indubitably living organisms, namely, the nerve cells. These are low-grade fellow-animals, but fellow-animals they are.[4] This fact has remained wholly external to the orthodox view of sensation. When it has been assimilated, must not the social view of sensation be the necessary consequence?[5]

There is a pronounced tendency, in present-day psychology, to stop short of this position, after having adopted premises that really imply it. Thus one writer tells us:

Conscious life is made of the same stuff that conduct is made of..... Focal consciousness consists of, is actually made of, the impulses that are in the process of becoming conduct..... The motive and the percept are not two different things. The percept is simply the more completely defined motive.[6]

Here we see a vigorous effort to conceive the active and the receptive aspects of consciousness as organically interrelated. Yet note the following reservation:

[4] "The body is a vast society of living cells" (C. K. Ogden, *The Meaning of Psychology* [New York and London, 1926], p. 36).

[5] See secs. 37, 39.

[6] L. L. Thurstone, *The Nature of Intelligence* (New York: Harcourt, Brace and Company, Inc., 1924), p. 12. Reprinted by permission of the publishers.

[There are] situations in which we relax and simply allow a sense-impression to register with an attitude of indifference on our part, .... The sense-impressions are focal and yet no action is in sight or even intended. I prefer to consider these volitionally indifferent mental states as slight ripples of the internal energy system caused by the stimulation of a receptor surface..... It is in that state that we can discriminate between sense qualities.[7]

It is not easy to see how a strictly "indifferent" ripple of consciousness, in which "*no* action is in sight or even intended," which yet is "focal," can be made consistent with the propositions that "focal consciousness consists of . . . . impulses . . . . in process of becoming conduct," and that "the percept is simply the more completely defined motive." This, at any rate, is clear: The author makes no attempt to show how his formulas could be used to explain sense data, in their qualitative differences from each other. He offers no suggestion as to how "redness," as part of the definition of a motive, differs from "blueness." Yet only such an attempt, successfully executed, could fully justify his doctrine. Furthermore, there seems but one way in which a sense datum could be regarded as a property of the subject's motive. There are only two ways in which a thing can be integral to a motive. One is as the motive's means.[8] But nothing can be mere means. A percept cannot be merely what it does or will do for us. Moreover, the sense datum is too objectively given, too definitely there in its own right, to be regarded so subjectively. The other relation to the motive is as its end, the intrinsic value which it recognizes, or in which it participates. Such an intrinsic value, in the form of "out-there-ness" characterizing the percept, can only be a socially intuited value, one which is the motive's end as a friend's enjoyment may be. The datum does not merely serve life but it also lives; it does not merely contribute to value or feeling, but it is feeling, socially objectified, endowed with "psychic distance." The "indifference" referred to by Mr. Thurstone is the detachment involved in this "psychic distance."

If the notion of objectified feelings, those intuited as out in

---

[7] *Ibid.*, pp. 130-31.

[8] "The psychiatrist would treat the environment as merely the means by which the patient seeks to express wants and cravings that are universal. This procedure is much more powerful and illuminating [than the usual one]" (*ibid.*, p. 17).

the extrabodily environment, seems shockingly ridiculous, I would ask that the actual experience of music, or of the "moaning" wind, be consulted, rather than some offhand mental reaction to the problem, and, further, that serious reflection be devoted to the question, how if social distance of emotions cannot be intuited it could ever be thought. In short, I point to the air of artificiality which infects the purely indirect theory of the consciousness of the social environment as such, an artificiality which many a thinker has felt though he perhaps could not produce adequate grounds for his conviction. That human neighbors are known almost exclusively through signs rather than directly is not here in dispute, but only the very different assumption that all neighbors are known only so. The fact is that the direct appearance of socially other emotional elements is all-pervasive in experience and needs only to be looked for with a little freedom from bookish and practical obsessions to be discovered as the manifest clue to the whole problem. We do not first project emotional qualities intuited as our own into an external organism, but rather a considerable part of the emotional content of experience is intuited from the outset as something coming from and qualifying the environing world in the first instance, and ourselves only derivatively or by participation. How far this intuition of objective feelings is an accurate awareness of the environment we need not here ask. (We pointed out above that the most immediate environment, the body, is a living one.) In any case, the general form of our imbeddedness in a social world—a form supposed to be a revelation exclusively of judgment or association or instinct operating upon sensory contents—is, in observable fashion, the very form of the contents themselves as contents, the form of their intuitive givenness. Thought and learning elaborate the details under this form, as in general the function of thought is not to produce the universal principles of experience, but to enhance the clear and effective grasp and control of the principles provided by the more primitive functions.

In his little book *The Psychology of Feeling and Attention*[9]—

[9] Pp. 291-92. Reprinted by permission of The Macmillan Company, publishers.

a model of scientific zeal and fair-mindedness—the late E. B. Titchener says:

> It is natural to suppose that the material of consciousness, the stuff out of which mind is made, is ultimately homogeneous, all of a piece. Let us make that supposition. The affections then appear .... as mental processes of the same general kind as sensations, and as mental processes that might, under favorable conditions, have developed into sensations. I hazard the guess that the "peripheral organs" of feeling are the free afferent nerve-endings .... and I take these .... to represent a lower level of development than the specialized receptive organ..... Had mental development been carried farther, pleasantness and unpleasantness might have become sensations.

But is it certain that they have not become just that? What is the taste of sweetness if not a pleasantness become a sensation? Almost the only thing overlooked by the distinguished psychologist is that the character separating "sense" from "feeling" is not chiefly any qualitative difference, but the manner in which the sense quality is localized in the body or externalized, projected out of it.

Among other merits claimed by Titchener for his theory is that it "explains the introspective resemblance between affections and organic sensations. Genetically, the two sets of processes are near akin; and it is natural that they should be intimately blended in experience."[10] This mode of inference, from genetic connection to similarity, is employed throughout biology and seems to me thoroughly sound. If men and monkeys were utterly different, no one would suppose a common evolutionary origin for them; and in spite of all that the emergent evolutionists have said, I do not see that the relationship of organs or functions within the same organism need be supposed an exception to this principle. That internal affection represents in some at least of its forms a less specialized and older mode of intuition than external sensation is scarcely doubtful. Now all evolutionary explanation views later-evolved functions as specializations of earlier. The business of the psychology of sensation should, therefore, be to exhibit its analogies with affection, its more primitive prototype. But the more these analogies are looked into, the more will the resultant picture of im-

[10] *Op. cit.*, p. 293.

mediate experience approach the pattern of the affective continuum. If Titchener failed to see this, it is partly because of his failure to note the logically indicated reversal of the proposition: Feelings are prototypes of sensation, into: sensations are specializations of feeling; with the implication that if the feeling prototypes are intuitions of value, the sensory specializations are not non-values, but only more developed value intuitions.

This analysis conforms to the facts of experience as some psychologists at least report them. Dashiell, for instance, has written:

> Forsaking the vast accumulation of petrified data piled up by the more intellectual operations of man for centuries and throwing ourselves .... into the heart of ordinary naïve human experience, we find ourselves in a world not so much of material objects .... as of weltering and striving, promising and threatening agents and forces..... These agencies are agencies that throw themselves as it were into our attention. They stand over against us in a genuinely objective sense—threatening, appealing, coercing, attracting, repelling. They appear as good, ugly, bad, magnificent, wrong, beautiful, upright. In fact, they are *just* these: they are goods, uglies, bads, magnificents, wrongs, beautifuls, uprights. As such and only as such are they there at all. The original material of all human experience presents itself in this intimate and face to face manner.[11]

I comment only upon the emphasized objectivity or "over against us" character of these affective tonalities, and upon the obvious relevance (brought out by the author himself) of this description to the problem of primitive animism. Is all experience, and not merely that of the savage, apart from the element of intellectual abstraction, i.e., of the performance of word habits, animistic in character?

However fantastic this may seem to many, they cannot refuse to consider the question just suggested, namely, whether it is reasonable to suppose that the notion of the world entertained by savages and children represents that world as in principle much more different from its actual appearance to the senses

---

[11] J. F. Dashiell, *Journal of Philosophy*, 1914, p. 492. (Reprinted by permission of the editors.) Wolfgang Köhler similarly says: "No one can hear naïvely the rumbling crescendo of thunder without understanding it as 'menacing.' .... What surrounds us in sensory space, we describe as restless or menacing or friendly, because these are the dynamical attributes or *Ehrenfels*-qualities which characterize the sensory experiences in question" (*Gestalt Psychology* [New York, 1929], p. 264).

than do the views of sophisticated modern intellects. Surely the primitive view would be more, rather than less, determined by sense experience in its concreteness. Intellectual advance has resulted not in a closer conformity of conceptions to the general quality of sense experience, but—a vastly different thing—in a gain in conformity to selected details, and particularly in the power to predict details. A vivid sense of what everyday experiences, on the whole, are like needs no science to impart, and it requires an immense training in abstractions to weaken or obscure it.[12] Still, even now we can recover the facts by experimental methods directed to this end. When we do so, we find ourselves confronted with the still insufficiently emphasized fact of objective feelings, feelings having the same locus in phenomenal space as sensory qualities, and indeed, according to a growing opinion, phenomenally one with the latter.

### SECTION 13. OBJECTIVE FEELINGS

A number of observers who have gone into the question with great care, detail, and skill have reached some agreement in regard to the real givenness of what they term the "characters" of colors or of sounds.[13] These are described as explicitly emotional and "anthropomorphic"; they constitute a sort of apparent personality of the sense quality in question, a mood or temperament intuited in it. This intuited inherence of character in the sense datum constitutes a problem, if we suppose the pure heterogeneity of the sensory and the character aspects. It appears to be rather generally accepted that those who insist that the character—e.g., the gaiety—is not really in the color or

[12] E. M. von Hornbostel says: "For us, alas, hearing and seeing, within and without, soul and body, God and the world, are divorced from each other. What as children we already knew, we are now seeking. Only old children—artists and wise men—know it still, see and hear still the life blooming everywhere about them" (*Melos*, IV, 294).

[13] See C. W. Valentine, *The Experimental Psychology of Beauty*. Also C. W. Valentine and C. Myers, "A Study of the Individual Differences in Attitude toward Tones," *British Journal of Psychology*, VII (1914), 68 ff.; Edward Bullough, "The Perceptive Problem in the Appreciation of Single Colors," *ibid.*, II, 406 ff., esp. pp. 433-48 and 459 ff., also "Psychic Distance as a Factor in Art," *ibid.*, V, 87-118; Charles Myers, *The Effects of Music*, ed. M. Schoen, chap. ii; Kurt Huber, *Der Ausdruck musikalischer Elementarmotive* (Leipzig, 1923), pp. 26-35; G. J. von Allesch, *Die aesthetische Erscheinungsweise der Farben* (Berlin, 1925).

sound are stating theory and not observation. Subjects insist and are clear that they see the character and the color in the same place, and as somehow one thing, a thing readily and radically distinguishable from their own reactive feelings or attitudes toward the external sense datum. They note frequently that the objective feeling may be in conflict with the observed reactive (intra-organic) feelings.

But there is this to be said. A considerable minority of subjects do not report "characters."[14] It is agreed that such subjects are found only among persons of little interest in or aptitude for aesthetic experiences. Still, they seem to exist. It appears to follow that, although characters when they are observed are observed in colors, yet, since the same colors are by some observed as lacking the characters, we must admit that color and its character are quite separable factors. How, then, can one appear to be really "in" the other? In answer it has frequently been suggested that the feeling has first been experienced in a more internal form and then "projected" unconsciously into the color. This process is admittedly unobservable, nor can observation reverse it and cause the character to leave the sense datum in order to relocalize itself within the body. The externality of characters is a stubborn and irreducible fact, so far as observation goes.[15]

Moreover, the projection theory must face the consideration, more and more accepted as an axiom by investigators into these problems, that when two things have no affinity or likeness it is impossible by any illusion to project one into the other. Into a few lines on paper we can project the meaning "house," but only because these lines have a genuine resemblance, however crude, to the actual shape of a house. The projected meaning fits and is homogeneous with that into which it is projected. Where this seems not to be the case, as in the printed word "house," the meaning is apprehended from but not projected

---

[14] Most of these subjects occur among those used by Bullough and Valentine; Huber and von Allesch seem to have found the character experience more nearly universally distributed.

[15] Cf. Huber, *op. cit.*, pp. 28-29.

into the word. In cases where, or in so far as, the projection occurs, there likeness will be found, if looked for sufficiently carefully. This is the principle which must be substituted for a mere indiscriminate projection of meaning upon an object regardless of its fitness to embody that meaning.[16] If colors have characters, they are like characters. If passions can be warm, then warmth has some trait in common with passion. Von Allesch has evolved a subtle theory according to which the factor in colors which is akin to the emotional life is the "dynamic" movement from one color to another. Thus, if orange is presented after yellow, there is a movement away from the yellow as the *niveau* of the experience, toward red as the "goal." The orange is a mere transition. This is ingenious and is also largely true. But the implication remains that whenever "warmth" of color feeling is intuited it is because the movement is toward red, and whenever it is gaiety that is felt, the movement is toward yellow. That is, the upshot of what is perhaps the most exhaustive study of the color experience in its qualitative essence ever made with modern experimental methods is that the old mystical doctrine that colors are manifestations of spirituality in specific phases is at least compatible with the facts. The most cogent objection to any such doctrine has hitherto been that sense quality and spiritual meaning or character can be independently varied. Von Allesch has unraveled part of the secret of this variability. After years of experiment he has demonstrated that any color can indeed be made the emotional equivalent of almost any other, but only in the following manner. It is possible, for example, to see yellow either as a cold or as a warm color, for red is warmer and green is colder. If, in other words, the *niveau* or standard of comparison (which need not be conscious) is red, yellow is cold; if the *niveau* is green, then it is warm. This is not speculation. Von Allesch was able to demonstrate the influence of the *niveau* in an impressively large proportion of cases. Furthermore, he showed that the movement from the *niveau* through the color to the goal beyond altered the color itself in the same direction as it did the emo-

---

[16] Von Allesch, *op. cit.*, pp. 41–43; Huber, *op. cit.*, pp. 32, 218 ff.

tionality.[17] A yellow which looks warm may be adjudged an orange; one which looks cold, a greenish yellow, etc.

Yet von Allesch's conclusion from this magnificent work is so cautious and so mildly at variance with traditional views as to appear almost insignificant.

Other theorists, recognizing the inadequacy of any ordinary association doctrine, and the difficulties in the way of "projection," still fail to venture upon a radical formulation of the issue.[18] What restrains them, apart from the weight of tradition, is doubtless the apparent independent variability of sensation and characters, and, above all, the fact that some subjects report the absence, in their experience, of the latter. I suggest that it is compatible with what we know of the control of introspection by habitual direction of interest to deny roundly that these failures to observe characters constitute strong evidence that the characters are not universally intuited. After all, to intuit is not the same thing as to be in a position, upon demand and without further ado, to know and report that we have so intuited. Those subjects who do not see the "characters" do not with equal intentness see the colors, and their protocols prove this through the preoccupation which they evidence with their own organic states and with various abstractions and distractions from the concrete datum itself.

According to the authors cited, the failure to see characters in colors or sounds occurs only with subjects whose aesthetic sensitivity is not marked, and in such cases the attention is divided between the sense qualities and (1) the subjects' organic state ("the infra-subjective type") or (2) abstract relationships of the sound or color to others of the same class of quality, i.e., brightness, pitch, or the like ("the objective type"), or, finally, (3) associations of the datum with other imagery ("associative type"). That (1) and (3) involve a diversion of attention is

---

[17] *Op. cit.*, pp. 34 ff., esp. p. 40. Huber's results with sounds are similar though necessarily more complicated (*op. cit.*, pp. 170–84).

[18] Huber, e.g., says that characters are "not further analyzable intermediaries" between sensations and feelings. The position of this book is that "not further analyzable" is an objectionably dogmatic expression for "I [or we] do not at present know how to carry analysis further."

manifest. That (2) also represents a failure to attain full attentional concentration upon the sensum is perhaps less clear. And yet, after all, the brightness of a red is not the redness in its full concrete character as given, but a highly one-sided consideration of the red together with simultaneous consideration of it in relation to other colors or to the whole scheme of colors; similarly with the consideration of tones in terms of pitch. The evidence thus implies that only the character-seeing observers found the sense quality itself sufficiently interesting to command the full focus of attention. It is taking a strange view of a datum of experience to suppose that only those who avoid focusing their attention upon it will see it as it is; and yet such is the case with sense qualities if they are really characterless. It is true that there is supposed to be a class of data which tend to conceal their true character when attended to. These are the emotions and feelings. But in the present instance the reverse seems true. It is those who attend as exclusively as possible to the sense data who see them as emotional tones, and it is those whose attention wanders to abstract considerations who seem not to be conscious of the tonality. The reader may urge, nevertheless, that it is persons of the "objective type" who see the datum as it is, since they alone report correctly upon its "objective" or real attributes (e.g., "pitch"), whereas the character seers indulge in obviously personal and fanciful descriptions. This contention, however, is not in accord with the facts. It is not true that neglect of the "character aspect" makes for more accurate observation of attributes. In the first place, the general correlation of "character type" with marked aesthetic appreciation points to an opposite conclusion; for in no class of persons is the accurate discrimination of attributes more developed than it is among artists or aesthetes. It has been found, moreover, that the most accurate matchers of colors are aware that they achieve this success by referring in their judgments to the emotional tone of the colors.[19] This is scientifically respectable evidence for two things: first, that it is the aesthetically minded,

---

[19] I. A. Richards, *Principles of Literary Criticism* (New York: Harcourt, Brace & Co., 1928), p. 99. Richards does not give the source of his statement.

those intent upon the emotional flavors of experience, who are the most accurate observers of its qualities, even those in its external sensory portions; second, that the qualities so observed are probably emotional in essence. If the most accurate observation of qualities as such proves to be interested in them as feelings, why should we strive to evade the natural implication that as qualities they are feelings?

The alleged independent variability of "sense" and objective "feeling," by which the distinctness of these concepts is often held to be demonstrated, comprises four possibilities:

1. The sensations sometimes exist without the feelings.
2. The sensations being constant, the feelings may vary.
3. The sensations varying, the feelings remain constant. (The discussion above of von Allesch's *niveau* doctrine is relevant to 2 and 3.)
4. The sensations being absent altogether, the feelings may occur. This is equivalent to saying that all the value of music could be had without the music.

Certainly, if any one of these could be proved, the affective theory of sensation would have been disproved. But the difficulties of such demonstration have been much underestimated. Propositions 1 and 4, being absolute negatives, are incapable of strict proof. The other propositions also offer serious difficulties. For instance, many who say that the same music feels very differently to different persons who nevertheless hear it alike would be surprised often to learn just how different the sense data in the two experiences actually are. Also most discussions of these matters pay scant attention to the all-important distinction between subjective and objective feelings.

In the interpretation of the latter the important question, too seldom discussed, is this: Can there be room in the same part of phenomenal space for two sets of qualities, sensory and emotional? Consider the visual field, for example. Can it contain, in one and the same area, colors, including their boundaries or shapes, and also, as an additional set of qualities, those of feeling tone? To me it seems an evident fact that colors and their spatio-temporal arrangements form a visual plenum, a logically saturated situation. What could be more impossible than the addition to this plenum of a whole set of emotional experiences localized in the same visual surface? If aesthetic properties are to be admitted in external experience, they cannot be admitted as additions to the sensory qualities, whose function is precisely to fill that portion of experience completely, endowing it with whatever qualitative determinations it is to have.

An exception to this principle might appear to be the simultaneous occurrence, in the same experiential place, of data from two senses—for example, a color and a sound, or a taste and a smell, or a temperature and a touch sensation. These pairs of qualities involve in each case equally concrete entities. Do they really appear at the same place without thereby losing their distinctness? This I cannot find to be the case. Where smell and taste, for example, cannot be intuited as in separate places or at separate times in the same place, there they cannot be intuited as qualitatively distinct; and so with all the other pairs. Moreover, as we saw in a previous section (6D), there is experimental evidence to confirm these conclusions.

Thus the rule is sustained that the occupancy of a certain portion of experience by a given sensory quality, say a color, constitutes the complete qualitative determination of that portion of experience. There is, therefore, in external experience, no further class of qualities, the aesthetic or tertiary, in such a portion. Since it is, nevertheless, an experimental result that tertiary qualities, "characters," appear in parts of phenomenal space occupied by sensory qualities, the inference is that these characters are the sensory qualities themselves, their constitutive natures—that, for example, the "gaiety" of the yellow is its yellowness.

The objection that the external localization of characters may be only an illusion is of doubtful relevance. For the real, as distinct from the apparent, locus of the characters is not in question. It is phenomenal or apparent, not physical, spatialization which is under discussion. Not that introspective reports of what appears are to be accepted as infallible; but that whatever error or illusion enters must be a matter of degree.

This is indeed the way of illusions generally. In dreams or hallucinations, for instance, we are not mistaken in believing ourselves to exist in a physical environment of certain general characters, but only in ascribing to this environment details which do not pertain to it. All the more must we be right in principle in imputing, on the basis of direct experience, emotional characters to extrabodily phenomenal space.

Much energy has been spent in efforts to interpret characters as illusory projections upon sense data with the object of rendering the facts about them compatible with the traditional materialistic view of sense qualities. These efforts have led to no generally accepted interpretation. Should not an effort now be made to determine whether the alteration of this traditional view in order to render it compatible with the experimental facts may not lead to a more satisfactory outcome?

### SECTION 14. IS FEELING AN ATTRIBUTE OF SENSATION?

The reality of objective feelings has led some psychologists to propose the acceptance of feeling as one of the "attributes" of sensory quality. This proposal, however, has met with little approval, and it is open to the following objections: (1) Feeling is itself subject to the attributes mentioned, and is therefore on a different logical plane from them. (2) Emotional content lacks the abstractness of the typical attributes by virtue of which they can subsist together in the concrete sense quality without competing with it for a place in experience. Emotional tone is "spread out" upon the sense object in the same concrete way as is, for example, the color itself; whereas the attribute of spatial or temporal extension is just the "spread-outness" itself; while the "intensity" is just the degree to which the quality spread out surpasses the threshold of noticeability, the degree to which it is something rather than nothing. The ascription of these factors to the sense quality does not complicate it as a reality but merely analyzes its status as real. As for "quality," this is simply that which distinguishes the sense datum occupying the given extension, with a given degree of vividness, from others which might have occupied it—in short, that which endows it with specificity or distinguishes it from being in its pure generality. What, then, is the function of tonality? Given definite distinction: (1) from mere nothingness (*intensity*); (2) from mere undifferentiated unity, the nothingness of the Parmenidean or Brahmanical One (*extensity* = simultaneous and successive plurality); (3) from the remaining species of being (*quality*), what further can be required? You may answer, tonality is needed in order to endow the datum with being-for-consciousness, regarded as a volitional and sentient as well as a purely cognitive entity. But in granting the intensity and quality of the datum as such, being-for-consciousness is already fully conceded; indeed, in granting being at all, being-for-consciousness, in *potentia* at least, is once and for all included, since what is is at least what we as minds can mean by this our concept of "being." That which we could not conceivably intuit, hence could not possibly imagine, is precisely that whose conception coincides with the conception of nonentity. Turn the question as one will, either the function of tonality is identically that of quality (or of one of its dimensions) or it has no function.

Or again, if feeling is conceived not as an attribute but as one or more of the dimensions of the attribute of "quality," then we must ask if this dimension (or dimensions) is additional to the ordinary dimensions (e.g., the three dimensions of the color solid) or is identical with one (or more) of them. The former alternative will scarcely recommend itself. It would mean that a certain shade, hue, and saturation of red could retain its brightness, hue, and saturation while varying in affective tone, and that this change would be a change in quality of the same logical type as the change from red to pink or purple. It would also mean that the notion of a redness sensation of determinate brightness, hue, and saturation, but indeterminate in affective tone, is a logical impossibility in just the same way as a redness without any particular hue or saturation. And, finally, it would indicate that the representation of color as three-dimensional is wrong; we should have a four- (or more) dimensional scheme. I wonder if a single psychologist believes that a fourth dimension so added would really refer to the same logical aspect (the qualitative, whereby the sense datum in itself differs from all other possible sense data otherwise than through spatio-temporal structure) as do the three generally conceded dimensions. Yet unless the doctrine that feeling is an attribute—a doctrine by no means without support in psychology—means this scarcely credible conception, there is only one other thing it can reasonably mean, viz., the affective continuum, according to which the dimensions of sensory quality are identically dimensions of affective quality.

Moreover, in so far as the facts compel the admission of objectified feelings, we have no choice but to find room somehow in the objective content of experience, that very portion, as we have just seen, so fully occupied by the sensory qualities, for a dimension or two of affective quality. We must face the issue and take our choice: the feelings are not intuited as in the sense datum, as objective, at all, or they are intuited as dimensions of sensory quality, coinciding with some or all of the recognized dimensions. The former view is forever irreconcilable with the factual experiences which motivate the many proposals to regard feeling as attributive or as somehow objective. The latter might perhaps enable us to do justice to the totality of standpoints, including Stumpf's theory, resting as it does upon unusually wide and careful observations, of feelings as sensations.

### SECTION 15. SUBJECTIVE FEELINGS

If attentive study of external sensations reveals their kinship to internal affections, it is also true that the close scrutiny of internal affections reveals their sensation-like character. In some of the most careful experimental studies of affective qualities yet assembled John P. Nafe reaches the following conclusion:

$P$ [pleasantness] in quality is a bright pressure, or quality lying between pressure and tickle. It is described as bright; sparkling; brilliant; active; like effervescence; . . . . dancing; shimmering; like points of light pressure; mild; misty; yielding; buoyant; . . . . fluffy; like the pressure component in warmth; like expansiveness of the body.

The quality of $U$ [unpleasantness] is that of dull pressure, or, according to some O's [observers], of a pressure between dull pressure and strain. It is described as .... drab; dead; rigid; less lively; somber; gloomy; more dense; heavy; sinking; thick; cold; hard; rough; harsh; grating; insistent; like bodily contraction.[20]

These results are, we are warned, to be regarded as valid "only under the conditions of the experiment." More work will doubtless need to be done. But, as they stand, the protocols clearly posit a sensation-like character for pleasantness-unpleasantness. "Pressure" is used, we are told, in a somewhat generalized sense, and it means having a quality like that common to the various cutaneous sensations. Not only are $P$ and $U$ thus compared to sensations, but they are often described as closely similar to the very sensations which are the objects of the feeling responses.

The softness [fur] was like the affection. There is something pressury and soft about the odor that is like $P$ itself.[21]
The sensory quality [a sound] is bright, more of the nature of the quality of $P$, it resembles $P$ much more than it does $U$.[22]
Not only did the two kinds of experience, sensory and affective, blend intimately, but they were very much alike.[23]

The lack of any radical qualitative gulf between sensation and affection could find no clearer statement.

What, then, was found to be the principal difference between feeling and sensation? The answer is easily read in the reports.

Somehow the sensory stuff is more sharply defined, coarser grained, and the affection is finer grained, looser. Also the affective part was pressury at the core, with arms running out that were bright, lively..... The affection was more like a background that the sensory stuff played over.....[24]
As soon as the affective part is the important thing, the sensory clings to that..... It melts in, is more intimately fused with the affective things, and yet stays qualitatively different, though beaten up. One can still say the two qualities are there, but the affection becomes the matrix which holds the qualities, whereas in the first part there are two matrices..... The character of affection is the prominence of the peripheral part rather than the central part. That seems to be rather constant.[25]
The odor quality became generalized. It seemed to take its character from the affective side rather than expressing its own character.[26]
It [the affection] covers the whole of experience.[27]

[20] "An Experimental Study of the Affective Qualities," *American Journal of Psychology*, XXXV (1924), 517. Reprinted by permission of the editor.

[21] *Ibid.*, p. 520.   [23] *Ibid.*, p. 520.   [25] *Ibid.*, p. 514.
[22] *Ibid.*, p. 518.   [24] *Ibid.*, p. 513.   [26] *Ibid.*, p. 513.   [27] *Ibid.*, p. 515.

From these quotations we see that subjective affection is recorded as less determinate but more enveloping than sensation, closer to awareness as a whole, to experience in the large. Sensation, conversely, is like particularized, objectified, parceled, clearly defined affection. The implication is that of the two factors the affective is the more primitive and fundamental, and the sensory a specialization of this primordial function. Thus between the two equations "feeling is a form of sensation" and "sensation is a form of feeling" there is reason in the protocols themselves to emphasize the latter. Nafe, however, seems interested solely in the former, partly because of the "tangible" character of the sensory aspect, its describability. He is anxious to avoid the scientifically nugatory result of having to dismiss affective quality as a not further analyzable qualitative variable. But then the same anxiety, applied to the sensory aspects, leads, as we have repeatedly seen, to the opposite result. Admitting that pleasantness—that is, immediate positive valuation—appears as a brightness, and its opposite as a dulness or darkness, what is this quality of brightness-dulness? In Nafe's account it appears intimately associated with intensity; but the relation of visual brightness to intensity has occasioned an as yet unterminated dispute, the satisfactory settlement of which depends, I should hold, upon the use, in the description of sensation, of the idea of valuation conceived as the central activity of mind. Thus the very motive which leads to the sensationalizing of the affective concept may lead to the affectivizing of the sensory concept.

In the excitement of the important facts brought out in Nafe's studies it would appear that the main problem has been almost lost sight of, the problem, namely, why pleasantness is a state of acceptance, of liking; and unpleasantness one of rejection or aversion. This problem now becomes that of explaining why liking is bright and disliking dull. Both this problem and that of the nature of brightness, in itself and in relation to intensity, may be resolved at one blow by an affective theory of sensory brightness. The sensory theory of affectivity leaves both aspects a mystery pure and simple.

It is true, however, that the mere application of the concept of affection, as ordinarily entertained, to the problem of sensory quality would accomplish little. For the minimum number of dimensions of such quality, additional to that of intensity, is two, whereas affection is usually defined as uni-dimensional. Upon this assumption it is indeed impossible that sensation should be a mere form of feeling.

There is, further, a troublesome paradox in Nafe's results. If pleasantness is brightness, all bright sensations should have a pleasantness affinity. Yet pain, whose affective affinity might be expected to be with unpleasantness, is described in other experiments conducted by the same investigator as distinctly bright. This outcome should be brought into connection with the admitted fact that pain is not always subjectively unpleasant. The problem is one to which we shall have to return (in sec. 34).

In the articles from which the material for this section was drawn there is a notable absence of the distinction between subjective and objective feeling. Nevertheless, the insistence in the protocols upon the pervasiveness of feeling, its immanence in the sensations, with which it is spoken of at times as "beaten up," shows that however the distinction between subjective and objective be drawn, feeling will transcend this distinction and force recognition of its presence on both sides of experience. This is also the conclusion of another investigator, who says: "We may safely say that feeling, i.e., pleasantness or unpleasantness, in itself, is neither subjective nor objective, but puts on the character of the global experience."[28] Of "objective feelings" the same author says: "From the descriptive point of view, the pleasant or unpleasant character appears to belong to the sensorial experience, as such; to be one of its properties; to constitute it, in the same way as the sensorial quality, properly so-called."[29] Experimental evidence is thus accumulating that sensation and affection are inseparable factors, with the

[28] G. B. Phelan, *Feeling Experience and Its Modalities: An Experimental Study* (London and Louvain, 1925), pp. 259–60.

[29] *Ibid.*, p. 255.

implication that we shall never understand either so long as we persist in regarding them as offering each a distinct problem for solution. There is but one problem, the qualitative dimensions of a pervasively affective experience with a subjective and an objective aspect.

### SECTION 16. ALLEGED CRITERIA OF THE DISTINCTNESS OF SENSATION AND FEELING

Among the factors which have enabled the division of mind into affective and non-affective elements or functions to become so deeply intrenched are some question-begging definitions.[30] For instance, one may say, and this in effect most psychologists have said, that feelings, like spatio-temporal configurations, are more abstract and general than the specific secondary qualities. Premissing the standard definition of feeling as degree of pleasantness-unpleasantness, it seems clear that these degrees have no such specificity as redness or sourness, since these two highly different qualities may coincide in degree of unpleasantness or its opposite. This doctrine of the uni-dimensionality of feeling is legitimate if it means that the term "affection" is to be reserved for the naming of degrees along the single contrast pleasant-unpleasant. In the same sense brightness is uni-dimensional; for it is just one among the variables of color experience. But it is another matter if it is said that "feelings," as concrete parts of experience (this pleasure, that suffering) differ from each other in only one way. This is like saying that colors differ only in their brightness. At least, feelings differ in one further respect—in their degree of objectification. And certainly, if enjoyment-suffering is inherently social, then several dimensions of variation are inevitable.[31] If research has failed to verify pro-

[30] The best discussion of this source of error, in its effects upon the interpretation of experimental results, is by J. G. Beebe-Center, in his valuable book, *Pleasantness and Unpleasantness*, chap. iii, esp. pp. 101-7. His distinction between feelings which cannot be objectified ("localized") and pleasant or unpleasant objects which can be localized is perhaps interpretable as an implicit admission of objective feelings. Certainly the distinction has much the same importance and function in his explanation of conflicting opinions as in that given in this section.

[31] See chap. vi. The multi-dimensional view has found renewed support in recent times. See, e.g., Kiesow in *Feelings and Emotions: The Wittenberg Symposium*, ed. C. Murchison (1928), p. 101; Müller-Freienfels, *Das Denken und die Phantasie*, pp. 21-23;

posals in this direction, this may show only the results of the uncriticized assumption underlying these researches, namely, the supposed non-social structure of immediacy.[32]

Another question-begging definition refers to feelings as experiences which are essentially vague, in contrast to the distinctness of primary and secondary qualities. Now, of course, experiences do fall into these two classes of the relatively vague and the relatively distinct, and if one wishes to reserve the word "feeling" for the former, one may do so. But one should then recognize, first, that since vagueness is a matter of degree, there is, at least as a matter of possibility, a continuum of qualities, uniting feelings and sensations in such fashion that the boundary between them is more or less arbitrary; and, second, that in employing the word "feeling" in this fashion one has left entirely open the question of the validity of that other dichotomy, the one dividing experiences essentially of an evaluatory or attitudinal character from those supposedly "neutral" in essence. The use of the word "feeling" to indicate both dichotomies must not lead to the prejudging of one on the basis of what has been proved only for the other.

A related circumstance which is often held to indicate a real difference between feeling and sensation is that it is characteristic of the former that attention to it reduces its intensity, and may even eliminate it from consciousness altogether; whereas attention to sensory contents is almost if not quite definable by reference to the increase in intensity and distinctness which accompanies it. This fact is held to be explained by the attitudinal character of feeling; for to feel is to assume an attitude of favoring or disfavoring, while to attend to and experience as an explicit datum or object is to abandon this type of attitude and to fall into the incompatible one of the mere spectator, whose first activity is to observe rather than to accept or reject, to re-

---

William M. Marston, C. Daly King, and Elizabeth H. Marston, *Integrative Psychology* (New York: Harcourt, Brace & Co., 1931); Burlton Allen, *Pleasure and Instinct* (New York: Harcourt, Brace & Co., 1930), p. 299; and especially Harlow and Stagner, "The Psychology of Feelings and Emotions," *Psychological Review*, XXXIX (1932), 570–89.

[32] Beebe-Center (*op. cit.*, pp. 60–67, 101–7) finds the question of multi-dimensionality still an open one.

cord rather than to evaluate. There is a plain and well-verified truth in this, and there is also, in subtle amalgamation therewith, an unproved and momentous assumption. This assumption is that to be immediately aware of an attitude means in all cases to have this attitude as one's very own, that all intuitions of appreciation are egocentric, that there is in immediacy no spiritual element of sympathetic participation by virtue of which a content may continue to be given as constituted by an attitude even while it is scrutinized as an object, and even though the attitude is not, except secondarily or by immediate sympathy, one's own.

It is not hard to see that the experiments which have been made to establish the fragility of feeling under the fire of attention have not been planned to deal with the validity of this non-spiritual assumption, but have relied upon that assumption as an unconscious axiom. The subjects are clear enough, I think, that the question before them is not whether the content continues, even under attention, to maintain a certain objective affective tonality, but only whether it continues to preserve its pleasantness or unpleasantness as determinant of their own satisfaction or dissatisfaction—in short, whether they continue to like or dislike, to enjoy or painfully endure, its presence. That there might be such a thing as the direct intuition of a liking or suffering given as that of another is not considered.

The significance of this neglect is brought out by recalling the experiments (sec. 13) upon the "characters" of colors or sounds. The joyousness or gloom of a color is here not, as a rule, apprehended as the subject's feeling or attitude, but as the feeling of the color, or of the colored object, to such an extent that the subject characteristically reports either that his own attitude or emotional state remains more or less in conflict with the objectified sensory feeling, or that by sympathetic participation in the latter there is induced in him a corresponding, though clearly distinct, subjective feeling. "The music sounded cheerful in parts .... but I felt in a contrary mood all the time"[33] is an example of such a report.

[33] Max Schoen (ed.), *The Effects of Music* (New York and London, 1927), p. 25.

The ability to maintain themselves under the scrutiny of attention is quite as characteristic of these objective feeling tones as is the corresponding inability of subjective or egocentric feelings. Indeed, a maximum of attention upon sensations themselves shows them to be feelings, to possess emotional qualities as their intrinsic essences. Any further feeling, distinct from the sensations and having them as objects, will be feeling about or toward feelings, an attitude toward attitudes—in short, the former feeling or attitude is social. The sensory feeling is objectified, and attention to it enhances it.[34] The only qualification required is one which applies to all immediate data in their relation to attention; namely, if attention means thinking about, analyzing, reflecting upon, then of course—whether the object so regarded is a sense datum or an emotion—the energy involved in the thinking process implies a diminution of that available for the sheer having of the immediate quality.

What is usually thought of as attention to sensations is merely a somewhat less ruthless subordination of them than ordinary to practical or intellectual reactions of which they are the mere springboard.[35] This is all very well when no great fineness of discrimination of the nature of the sense datum is required; but when there is need of maximal and prolonged attention, there is only one way to get it: by falling, deliberately or not, into an attitude of pliancy and emotional hospitality—in short, as we shall see in detail later, an aesthetic attitude.

Thus, the true dichotomy suggested by the proposed criterion is not between feelings and sensations, but between egocentric and altercentric pleasantness-unpleasantness.[36]

Another fashion in which the genus feelings might by defini-

[34] When Külpe says, "Feeling has too little objectivity . . . . for the attention to be directed and held upon it" (quoted by Titchener, *op. cit.*, pp. 70–71), he is making a relatively true statement about the more subjective feelings, but not about the most objective species of feelings, i.e., on our view, the sensations.

[35] "Attention has an essentially disintegrative function" (A. O. Oeser, "Experiments on the Abstraction of Form and Color," *British Journal of Psychology*, XXII, 4, 318). See also his "Tachistoskopische Leserversuche," *Zeitschrift für Psychologie*, CXII (1929), 139 ff.

[36] This view seems to be confirmed by the excellent discussion by Beebe-Center (*op. cit.*, pp. 91–95).

tion be made to exclude sensation is the following. Feeling as a sense of good and evil, as pleasantness and unpleasantness, seems to imply a positive or negative, an accepting or rejecting, reaction of the organism. Now if feeling is a reaction of the organism as a whole, we are at least tempted to think of it as, at any moment, the total reaction of the organism at that moment to the sum of ingredients in its experience, including its sensations; but clearly there can be but one total reaction at a time, and clearly a given sensory quality is not that total reaction. This inference, however, is a *non sequitur* from the doctrine that feeling involves the total organism, since all consciousness does that, and since there is a clear and necessary distinction between reaction of the whole and the whole of such reactions. In an organism there are no reactions not of the whole, so that if there can be more than one process at a time, then there can also be more than one action of the whole. As a fact, investigators are less wedded now than they were to the doctrine of only one affectivity at a time, no agreement in its favor having been attained and many careful experimenters in quite diverse fields having found the structure of affection in terms of subordinate or conflicting simultaneous affections to be an evident and practically indispensable conception.[37] Certainly if feeling can ever be immediately social (feeling of feeling), then the doctrine "one feeling at a time" cannot be true.[38]

There is one further criterion of affection in distinction from sensation: feeling involves an "opposition" of positive and negative, liking and disliking. Does sensation exhibit a similar polarity? I think the answer is that in whatever sense feeling falls into opposites, sensation does so likewise. It is, as we have seen (in sec. 5C), precisely in terms of polarities that the facts of sensation are to be described. The failure so to describe them involves, in fact, some incurable self-contradictions. Some psychologists hold, however, that wherever polar opposition is found in experience, say in relations of color discord, this is due

---

[37] See, e.g., H. Henning, *Der Geruch*, p. 42; Phelan, *op. cit.*, pp. 255, 284–86.

[38] Beebe-Center concludes that "it is possible for a pleasant object and an unpleasant one to be experienced simultaneously" (*op. cit.*, p. 90).

to feeling.[39] This argument, like so many others, favors the separation of sensation and (objective) feeling only if the separation is already presupposed. I should agree that color opposition is a conflict of color affections; I should not agree that these color affections are other than the color sensations, and as partial proof I should adduce the very polarity in question.[40]

### SECTION 17. HOW FEELINGS BECOME SENSATIONS

The proposition that sensation is what feeling becomes when externally localized in phenomenal space implies a process of objectification which should be capable of experimental detection. Relevant experiments have in fact been made, and with results which confirm the hypothesis. Bichowsky, for example, reports his findings as follows:

> The first[41] conscious effect that can be traced to a stimulus of the sense-organs is a feeling which does not possess spatiality or temporal quality..... Such feelings or pre-sensations, as they will be called ...., have emotional tone and feeling quality..... They differ with the kind of stimulus, but this difference is not describable except by incomplete figures of speech. They were said to have "emotional tone." "They were an emotional tone spreading over the whole consciousness." "It felt cold" (the 'pre-sensation' blue)." "It was not, however, the cold 'feel' due to a cold stimulus." "The feels of (green and of the taste of cream) were both soothing and smooth and of about the same intensity but they were not alike."
> "The 'feel' was unstable and tended to generate the sensation." "It acted as a stimulus." "It disappeared, the sensation took its place." "There was a closing in of the feel, followed by a sudden perception of position and shape. The feel still remained, however, as a background on which the new perception arose." "I can always feel the coming sensation—sometimes though I have the feel of a visual something without the perception of position or shape."[42]

---

[39] Titchener, *op. cit.*, pp. 56–61.

[40] See secs. 5C, 20, 32. Titchener held that black and white are opposite only as zero and maximum intensity, and hence not, like pleasantness-unpleasantness, as involving an indifference or neutral point. But he also held that the difference between black and white is qualitative and not merely one of intensity. Now this qualitative difference turns out, upon investigation, to involve just such an indifference point. See sec. 32.

[41] This "first" is meant in a literal and accurate sense. Another author says that the "character" aspect of sounds is on the average the first to be reported, one half to one second being the average time required for this report (Huber, *op. cit.*, p. 30).

[42] F. Russell Bichowsky, "The Mechanism of Consciousness: Pre-sensation," *American Journal of Psychology*, XXXVI, 588–96.

By scanning the rest of this remarkable article one sees that the only unambiguous difference noted between the "emotional tone" of the pre-sensation and the character of the sensation proper refers to the degree of distinctness of the spatio-temporal configuration. We stand here upon a great divide of thought. Turn one way, and down a swift incline we soon reach the position—sensations are objectified (spatialized) affects (this spatialization being itself, I hold, nothing but the social character inherent in emotion itself). Turn the other way, and we fall back into the traditional—sensations are sensations. Which way leads to the truth? One thing is sure, the passages quoted above are not hopelessly eccentric; results apparently consistent with them have been attained by careful experimenters both in this country and in Europe.[43]

According to Spearman, four different methods have confirmed the hypothesis that sense data are externalized subjective states, only relatively distinguishable from the "self."[44] Perhaps Jaensch's work on "eidetic" phenomena, midway between phantoms and perceptions, is also to be considered here.

### SECTION 18. THE PERSISTENCE OF ASSOCIATIONAL AND FACULTY PSYCHOLOGIES

Psychology seems to be passing from a stage in which the basic principle of intelligible relationship among its data was the law of association—conceived as a superficial connection among elements otherwise profoundly distinct in nature and being—to a stage in which associative phenomena are seen as secondary results of a more intimate union, a veritable integration by which elements are intrinsically qualified through their relevance to one another.[45] The first conception regards mere existential togetherness as the key to mental events. The second

---

[43] Bichowsky did not describe his technique, but confirmatory results, without this deficiency, are given by R. B. Catteil in his monograph, *The Subjective Character of Cognition and the Pre-sensational Development of Perception* ("British Journal of Psychology Monograph Supplements," No. XIV), esp. pp. 74-77; and by G. B. Phelan, *Feeling Experience and Its Modalities* (London and Louvain, 1925), p. 255.

[44] C. Spearman, *The Nature of Intelligence*, chap. xiv, and *Creative Mind*, chap. xi.

[45] See Georges Dwelshauvers, *Traité de psychologie* (Paris), pp. 103 f.

emphasizes essential constitutive interrelatedness, i.e., partial identity, and therefore also similarity. It is a sign that the transition is not yet complete that the indications which universal experience provides of qualitative analogies between modes of sensation, or between sensation and feeling, are still brushed aside under the head of pure associations. If associations (relations not grounded in the natures of the entities) are secondary phenomena, then it is precisely evidences of intrinsic relationships, signs of a common life pervading all the mind, and of the affinities by which this life, in its identity, is revealed—it is precisely evidences of this sort which we must seek, and which we must discredit only as the facts compel us to do so. But it cannot well be denied that the prevailing attitude is the opposite of this, all hints of similarities being considered provisionally as associational in origin, if there are even a few facts (and of course there nearly always are) to render this view prima facie plausible. Associations are regarded as practically proved upon an amount and quality of evidence which would be brushed aside as absurdly inadequate if offered as proof of similarity. This attitude was logical when association ruled psychology. With the open rebellion in principle against this rule the attitude becomes a mere anachronism doubtless due chiefly to the fact that sensory problems are no longer in the center of interest.[46]

Similar remarks apply to the abandonment of "faculty" psychology in principle, and the adherence to its implications in detail. What is sensation, in the current acceptation of the concept, but a faculty, totally distinct from that other faculty of feeling; and, indeed, what is the doctrine of modes but a set of faculties? Sensation cannot feel, nor can it give us anything comparable to a feeling; hearing cannot see, nor can it give us anything in the least like color. After all, a faculty has always meant simply a power or capacity, a potency, so that the only intelligent objection to the concept is on the score of the ex-

[46] That association is a real and important law I do not deny; the contrary of this denial follows from the organic or social theory of feelings set forth in this book. I am insisting only that similarity is an equally fundamental aspect of the organic unity which is mind. Or, if you prefer, association may be by resemblance as well as by contiguity, and the latter presupposes the former.

aggerated distinctness sometimes assumed between the different capacities. This is the phase of the doctrine which is most reluctantly abandoned. So much easier is it to change our words than our thoughts, so much easier is it to despise a term than to reform a concept!

### SECTION 19. ATOMISM IN PSYCHOLOGY

Among the antiquated modes of thought not yet wholly eradicated from psychology is a certain species of atomism. As applied to the theory of sensation, this doctrine implies that certain of the sense qualities are complexes of which others are the simple units. Thus some qualities are, as it were, molecules, and others are atoms. Two radically different levels of logical complexity, that is, are held to be involved. Now there is, in fact, just one sense in which such difference of complexity can genuinely be verified in experience. This sense is spatial; for example, a patchwork of different colors seen as such is complex compared with the unit color areas of which it is composed. Simplicity is identifiable as homogeneity throughout a spatial extent; complexity, as heterogeneity of quality in distinguishably different portions of space. The complexity of tones and overtones is of this character. When the overtones are distinguished, they are found not to coincide in auditory space. The mere fact that they seem "higher" or "lower" has been shown to involve spatial difference.[47] On the other hand, the alleged complexes of vision, such as orange, do not present spatial heterogeneity, in every distinguishable portion of the phenomenon the same quality of orange being observed. Wherein, then, consists the complexity?

Brentano has an ingenious answer. The heterogeneity of orange, he says, is spatial, but the qualitatively different portions —some pure red, some pure yellow—of which it is composed are too small to be individually distinguishable.[48] The objection is that this hypothesis is descriptively irrelevant. As we see it, the

[47] See sec. 6B. Inasmuch as an odor-pitch has recently been discovered, the same principle may be assumed to apply to olfactory mixtures (Troland, *Sensation*, p. 279).

[48] Franz Brentano, *Untersuchungen zur Sinnespsychologie* (Leipzig, 1907), p. 18.

§ 19   CONFLICT OF OPINIONS IN PSYCHOLOGY   139

color is a homogeneous expanse, which as homogeneous is seen to have certain relations to other colors, such as red and yellow. If, then, an indiscernible heterogeneity is proposed as explanation of the redlikeness and yellowlikeness of orange, the answer is that a complete explanation is possible which does not involve this assumption. A dimensional analysis of color shows, as we have seen (sec. 5C), that the variables required for this alternative explanation are in any case unavoidable, so that the proposed additional factor of heterogeneity is without excuse. But Brentano and others urge that direct intuition shows heterogeneity. To the objection that many deny this intuition Brentano urges that everyone uses expressions, such as "yellow-green," which imply the mixture conception. Yet Brentano himself points out that we use phrases like "northwest" without meaning, let us say, that a northwest wind is a mixture of a north and a west wind. Thus he grants, rather in spite of himself, that the mere fact that the description of something involves complexity does not unambiguously indicate the complexity of the thing described. But, he argues, the fact that in some cases we are quite clear that this is so, whereas in the color instance we tend to regard the complexity as objective, shows that this instance is of a different kind. This reasoning overlooks the fact that spatial geometry is easier to grasp than nonspatial applications of geometrical principles. We do not suppose a man of medium height to be a mixture of a giant and a dwarf, as some suppose gray to be a mixture of black and white, because in the former case the structural relations in question are so directly apprehended through the intuition of space. In the latter case, where the relations have no immediately spatial character, the inevitable tendency is to look for a spatial analogy. Two forms of this analogy are available. According to the one, black and white are as the ends of a line, and gray as the series of points constituting the interior of the line. In other words, there is one variable with two extreme and numerous intermediate values. According to the other, black and white are as atoms and grays as molecules—that is to say, the latter consist of parts somehow analogous to the spatial divisions of matter. The dimensional relations formulated in the previous analogy are then deduced as corollaries from this atomic analysis. Since atomic analysis is the greatest single discovery of natural science, it is not strange that the attempt should be made to apply it to every problem, and to the problem of sensory qualities all the more because of the tempting suggestiveness of the fact that such qualities may indeed result from combinations of stimuli, as in pigment mixture. It remains true that such non-spatial atomic analysis is a logical monstrosity. It is the very meaning of space that it, and it alone, is the form of simultaneous combination of factors capable of separate occurrence, in the sense in which such combination is here in question.

The tendency to slip uncritically into the physical analogy is well shown in the following argument: "A blue-green may approach so very near to pure green as to be barely distinguishable from it, so that the casual observer would regard it as a pure green. It seems strange to say that such a blue-green contains no green at all."[49] The strangeness depends wholly upon the assumption that likeness means identical parts, which is the question at issue.[50] This assumption is insinuated through the metaphorical expression "pure." The metaphor is justified to the extent that mixture of elements does imply resemblance between the products of such mixture and its elements; but the conversion of this into the proposition that one of the terms of a resemblance must be a simple element of the other is a *non sequitur*.

It might be objected against our account of atomic qualitative analysis that no one can really have had the physical analogy in mind, since to describe, say, the difference between one orange and another we must evidently conceive the quantities of red and yellow in the mixture to vary, so that the presence or absence of these simple qualities is not an atomic affair. To this I answer that I cannot believe that any consistent conception

---

[49] G. F. Stout, *Manual of Psychology* (1899), p. 149. This paragraph is not in 3d ed.

[50] See von Kries, *Allgemeine Sinnesphysiologie* (Leipzig, 1923), pp. 124-30, for a careful analysis of this assumption.

whatever underlies the notion of non-spatial qualitative mixtures, and that there seems clearly to be an uncritical blend of true atomism with vaguer common-sense ideas, such as that of water as a spatially homogeneous mass which can be used in any arbitrary amounts to adulterate liquids. If there is in modern science a more uncritical notion than that of amounts of yellow in orange, I should be glad to be told of it.

Stout's argument might be parodied as follows: "Two twins have faces so much alike as to be barely distinguishable from each other. It seems strange to say that face A contains no amount of face B at all." It is worth noting too that we might speak here also of purity, as of a pure Roman nose, without thinking of the outline of an impure nose as the outline of a pure one plus a certain quantity of the outline of another type of nose, also conceivable in pure form. We leave it to Stout (who may well have changed his mind since writing his manual) to say which twin's face is simple and which complex, and pass on to note that Stout very honestly concedes that blue and green are not literally components of blue-green.

> What is probably in the mind of those who deny the combination of blue and green is that a blue-green cannot be simply defined as blue+green. The components by entering into so intimate a combination are modified in a peculiar way. This modification is a new element which may be regarded as simple..... But the components abstractly regarded are not the less discernible as partaking of the nature of blue and green (*loc. cit.*).

Thus we have as the modified mixture conception this: blue-green is so describable because it contains something resembling (a "modification" of) blue and something similarly resembling but not identical with green. The question remains: By what right do we call these somethings blue and green, even if we add the question-begging phrase "abstractly regarded"? The modification of blue into the corresponding component of blue-green is said to be simple, and hence inexplicable, but would it not be simpler still and more candid to accept the resemblance of blue-green to its two neighbors as ultimate, instead of pretending to analyze it in such an unintelligible fashion? On the other hand, to hold that blue and green are discernible in blue-green in *un*-

modified form seems to me scarcely honest. Certainly the fact must be faced that many excellent psychologists have totally lacked the consciousness of such a capacity.

The one real basis for Stout's view is given in his remark that "the *respect* in which blue and blue-green resemble each other .... is different from the *respect* in which green and blue-green resemble each other..... This appears to me a sufficient reason for inferring complexity in the blue-green." This inference is correct, but it gives no support whatever to the notion that these respects are blue and green themselves. And the fact that blue and green are taken as reference points for description in preference to blue-green is also explicable without supposing that they are any simpler than the latter, just as north and east are no simpler than northeast, although more natural units in description. Nothing could well be clearer than that the suppressed premiss of Stout's, Brentano's, and every other argument known to me for the mixture view is the rejection, without a hearing, of the possibility of a dimensional rather than atomic analysis of sensory qualities. The only important question is unconsciously begged throughout. This is not surprising, considering the one-sidedly atomistic character of all modern science prior to the present century.

That the conception of qualitative simplicity has not produced scientific results has been rather widely admitted. As Nafe declares, "There is no known criterion for simple qualities except the impossibility of psychological analysis, and there is no agreement as to which experiences are analyzable. Some authors posit three simple qualities of skin sensations, others more than thirty, although convincing reasons for such categories are lacking."[51] Surely "impossibility" has here no useful meaning, since the capacity of each psychologist to analyze qualities into others is proved to be different from that of almost every other. There is, I dare say, no quality whatsoever that some recognized contributor, or several, to psychological science has not, to his own satisfaction, analyzed, nor any that others

[51] In Murchison, ed., *Foundations of Experimental Psychology*, p. 400.

have not found themselves unable to analyze. The criterion is thus subjective and hence scientifically of little or no value.

There is, however, a second type of psychological atomism which, though less popular, is, I believe, more worthy of respect. The peculiarity of this type consists in its application of atomic analysis impartially to all sensory qualities, however primary or fundamental. An early example is Leibniz. To the Lockian contention of the simplicity of sense qualities, Leibniz replies that this simplicity consists only in our inability to detect in sensory impressions the "minute perceptions" of which they are subconsciously composed. These "minute perceptions .... form I know not what, these tastes, these images of the sense qualities, clear in the mass, but confused in the parts, these impressions which surrounding bodies make upon us, which involve the infinite, this connection which each being has with all the rest of the universe. ...."[52] This conception of subconscious parts of our conscious perceptions has had many echoes in recent thought. Part of its strength lies in the example which physics offers of the power of atomistic analysis. This power is not destroyed by the new physics, for a relativized atomism is now as important as absolute atomism formerly was. But at least two doubts arise. First, many will tell us that a sensation as such, as a conscious fact, is only what it is given as, and contains as parts only what it actually seems to be divided into. Observation, being here the definition of the thing observed, is infallible. This seems to me a meaningless doctrine. If it were true, then the act of observation might be as careless as one pleased; it could not go wrong. Or, if it could go wrong, then it is to be presumed that it would always err in some minute degree or other. Absolute accuracy is an infinite ideal, except in pure mathematics. And surely also vagueness is, sometimes at least, a fact of our perception. And what is this vagueness if not an imperfect apprehension of whatever it is that we directly apprehend? How convenient it would be if introspection were indeed infallible! Granting its fallibility and its vagueness, then the imperceptible

---

[52] *New Essays*, ed. Langley, p. 48.

atomic parts spoken of might be there in spite of their imperceptibility.

The second objection to this type of atomism is that its expounders have not yet taken to heart the relativity inherent in the new atomic concept, have not yet seen that while it is a partial explanation of many phenomena it is an adequate explanation of none. They have tried to use it to explain features which only a wave-concept, as it were—only a concept of variations in a continuous medium with specified dimensions—can properly account for. Consider, for instance, the following from Herbert Spencer:

> If the unlikenesses among sensations of each class may be due to unlikenesses among the modes of aggregation of a unit of consciousness common to them all; so, too, may the much greater unlikenesses between the sensations of each class and those of other classes. There may be a single primordial element of consciousness.[53]
>
> It is possible that something of the same order as that which we call a nervous shock is the ultimate unit of consciousness.[54]

Some similar notions have been expressed more recently.[55] And it cannot be denied that the new all-or-none law gives striking support to the hypothesis. It is physiological fact that differences in the patterning of an at least approximately identical form of nervous shock are the conditions of all the variety of sensations. The trouble is that so far no one has succeeded in actually explaining in this fashion the particular differences which we find among sensations. The theory remains in the general program stage. And, on the face of it, difference in the "mode of aggregation" seems a far cry from such a difference as that between red and yellow. Yet there are some striking possibilities. The example often used of the quality of smoothness as due to the blending-together of rapidly and regularly succeeding nerve pulses throws light on both auditory and cutaneous sensations. Indeed, one can even feel something smooth about certain colors, and it may not be an accident that it is the short wave-lengths of which this is true, whereas it is the long or red

---

[53] *Principles of Psychology*, I, 150.   [54] *Ibid.*, p. 151.
[55] See, e.g., C. A. Strong, *The Origin of Consciousness* (London, 1918), pp. 303–22; Strong, *Essays on the Natural Origin of the Mind* (London, 1930), chap. ii; Durant Drake, *Mind and Its Place in Nature* (New York, 1925), pp. 118–31.

waves which are rough (see Pikler's view as presented in the next section). There is also no difficulty in explaining brightness-intensity through the temporal spacing of pulses. Still, there seems to be more in the differences of color and sound and emotion than all such conceptions could hope to cover.[56]

Since in physics it is radically untrue that modes of aggregation of particles form the complete explanation of anything, since particles must be interpreted in terms of waves in a continuous medium, surely we have even less reason for expecting the atomic view to prove sufficient in psychology, where more than elsewhere the whole seems to dominate over the parts, as well as to be a resultant of their separately computable activities. The view justified by scientific logic is that the modes of variation characterizing mind as a living responding organism will throw at least as much light upon the individual units of which this organism may be conceived to consist as the modes of aggregation of the latter will throw upon the observable gross variations. We must seek the dimensions of mind as such. These dimensions, like those of space-time in the smallest physical particles, are probably found even in the action of the unit nerve cells, which also are organisms. Herein lies the significance of the tendency among the atomistic psychologists toward panpsychism, a significance which can never be seen so long as the basic dimensions of experienced qualities remain unclarified and so long as it is supposed that the atomic psyches are entirely exempt from these dimensions, so that the atoms of pain, for example, are conceived as quite devoid of a painlike quality. In that case their natures would escape all imagining to such a degree that the charge of unscientific mysteriousness, or even meaninglessness, so often made against panpsychism would be quite justified. The dimensions of the macrocosm are not absent in the microcosm; the basic modalities of life are in all that lives and all that composes the living being.[57]

[56] If they have any truth, these conceptions break down the absolute dichotomy of structure and quality upon which rests the doctrine that one cannot know if others experience the same qualities as one's self (see sec. 4).

[57] Cf. J. Pikler, *Schriften zur Anpassungstheorie des Empfindungsvorganges*, No. 4, p. 271.

## SECTION 20. DIMENSIONAL THEORIES OF SENSATION

The tradition which furnishes the requisite balance or complementation to the atomic view of qualities is at least as old as Aristotle. According to this thinker, sense qualities are not ineffable, but display a certain polarity by means of which they may be described, and in terms of which also their connection with physical conditions may be explained. Bitter, said Aristotle, is privation of nutrition in food—and this, on the whole, is the fact. But bitter is privative psychologically, decidedly negative as an objective feeling tone (whatever positive reactive feelings may sometimes attend it). So also with black and white; the former is the privation of seeing, and psychologically it well expresses this fact. The remaining colors embody related differences, in a manner which Aristotle did not make particularly clear. In the *Farbenlehre* of Goethe an attempt was made to carry out this Aristotelian interpretation with detailed thoroughness; but since more recent attempts of the same nature, embodying the enormous advance in factual knowledge achieved since Goethe's day, are open to our consideration, it is unnecessary to discuss the success or failure of Goethe's efforts.

Among contemporary psychologists, Julius Pikler seems to have made the most thorough investigations into the possibility of a dimensional—that is, a genuinely explanatory—account of sensory quality. In spite of Pikler's astonishing originality, the essential mark of his theory is little more than the completeness with which he carries out tendencies almost universally accepted, as general principles, in present-day psychology. His is, in fact, the only theory of sensation known to me in which the general revolt against the materialistic categories of the last century becomes complete.

In outline, Pikler's "adaptational" theory is as follows:[58]

1. Qualitative differences are not due to atoms of quality, miraculously present in the soul and no less miraculously combined into complex or molecular qualities; they are expressions of dimensions, continuous variables, of the adjustment of life

---

[58] *Ibid.*, Nos. 1 and 4.

to its environment. The relation between primary and non-primary qualities is not that of simple to complex—"Orange is not red and yellow, but *neither red nor yellow*, it differentiates itself from red in the direction of yellow, from yellow in the direction of red."[59] Primary qualities represent extreme values of variables which are present in intermediate degree in the secondary qualities; the former are "limiting qualities" (*Grenzqualitäten*), the latter, "intermediate qualities" (*Zwischenqualitäten*).

2. The supreme law of sensory response is the self-preservative tendency of the organic being. Confronted with a change in the environment, a stimulus, to remain essentially itself in and through this change is the problem of which the sensory response is the solution. The quality of the response varies with the more special form of the problem and is explicable by reference to the latter.

3. All response has three attributes: extensity, protensity, and intensity. In each attribute there are configurations (Gestalten): in the first, spatial forms, in the second, temporal rhythms; in the third, qualities. Qualities are the modalities of intensity. Intensity is the key to all qualities as space is the key to all shapes.

4. The organism is adapted, at any one time, to a certain midvalue of intensity. What falls below this is either "dark" (also "dull") or else "empty" (e.g., silence, as usually responded to); what exceeds it is sharp, bright, or full of life. If there is no other complication, such differences of brightness or sharpness or fulness will exhaust the phenomenon, and we shall have unsaturated or "toneless" qualities like the grays or mere pressure sensations. If, however, there is a dual response to the intensity of the stimulus such that the adaptations to both low and high intensity occur simultaneously in a certain conflict with each other, then saturated qualities, such as colors in the narrower sense, arise. This dual response varies independently in two ways, and thus there are two dimensions of saturated qualities. If put into Cartesian form, these dimensions may be char-

[59] *Ibid.*, No. 4, p. 231.

acterized as those of *conquest* and *balance*. The four extremes are as follows. If an incipient bright response is opposed and overcome by a dull response, that is negative conquest. Example, blue. If an incipient dull response is opposed and overcome by a bright response, this is positive conquest. Example, yellow. If an incipient bright response is opposed and held at bay but not crushed by a dull response, this is negative balance. Example, green. If an incipient dull response is similarly checked, but not crushed by a bright response, this is positive balance. Example, red. Non-primary qualities are simply intermediate values of the same variables. Thus orange is halfway between positive balance and complete positive conquest.

Evidence for the doctrine is found first of all in the directly observable characters of the qualities. Thus red and green, the two balance colors, agree in being neither bright nor dull; but they differ in that the negative balance color, green, is gentle, "harmless," whereas red, the positive, is "rough," active. Again yellow is not simply bright, but in contrast to white has a "piquancy" in its sharpness which the sheer brightness of white lacks. Other evidence is seen in the Perkinje phenomenon, in the possibility of color vision with neutral stimulus, and in the ready explanation furnished of complementation—naturally positive and negative conquest, or balance, neutralize each other.

In all senses where saturated qualities occur, the same variables are found. Positive conquest—called "sharpness"—is characteristic of yellow, salt, burning, and itch, in vision, taste, smell, and touch, respectively. Negative conquest—mildness—is common to blue, sweet, flowery, and stroking (contact with fur, for example). Negative balance—tartness (*Herbheit*)—yields green, sour, vinegary, tickle. Positive balance—roughness—gives red, bitter, foul, and pain.

In non-saturated sensations the parallel is to the grays, except that the equivalent of blackness is lacking wherever absence of stimulation is not sharply attended to as such. Pikler's discussion of black seems to me greatly superior to all others in print, and of itself to entitle him to more attention than he has received.[60]

So much for the parallelism of the senses. What of the differences?

5. Pikler holds that differences between the senses are intelligible with reference to the nature of the stimulus. Thus pressure sensations express the crude mechanical character of the stimulating force; odors also give us a sense of force acting upon us but one of a much subtler, more delicate kind; while tastes are intermediate, cruder than odors, finer than pressures. Thermal sensations give an impression of expansiveness and contraction corresponding to the immediate effect of heat upon the tissues. Sound and color embody wavilinear forces, whose character is that their actuating cause reverses its movement periodically, i.e., it counterbalances, neutralizes, in this sense nullifies, itself. Hence sound and light seem curiously insubstantial. Yet with a difference—for sound, though not like a substance to us, seems yet crude and material compared to color.

6. The relation to the stimulus also explains the differences within each sense. Thus sweet gives a sense of harmony with the activity of the organism; sour and salt and bitter, ever greater disharmony; similarly with stroking, tickle, itch, and pain. These relations of harmony or its opposite are held to obtain objectively, physiologically. Again low notes are dull, heavy, gloomy because their stimulus is too lethargic to bring the organism into full activity, but massive and hence productive of voluminous or diffuse though weak response. High notes are intense, ethereal, but thin for inverse reasons.

7. The explanation of all such correspondences[61] is that the organism tries to preserve its own rhythms in the face of the external changes impinging upon its receptor organs, and in thus counteracting, neutralizing such changes, it produces responses which duplicate the pattern of the latter.

[60] *Ibid.*, pp. 169-97.

[61] Do these correspondences not suggest an affirmative answer to the question discussed in sec. 4 concerning the objective describability of sense qualities?

This is the first well-developed theory of the sense qualities as intelligible facts yet to be presented. However erroneous this theory may prove to be, it is certainly an honor to have opened practically a new province to scientific explanation. The only criticism I wish here to suggest is that, on the physiological side, no use appears to be made of the important all-or-none law.

The dimensional approach to sensory quality has found defense in a form less disturbing to current intellectual fashions, at least to those obtaining in the United States, as an incident in the development of what its originators entitle "integrative psychology."[62] Its basic tenet is that consciousness is nervous integration and that modes of consciousness are therefore modes or patterns of such integration. Sensory qualities are one class of such patterns, emotions are another; but for all integrations certain general possibilities are relevant. These constitute the universal forms of conscious life. Moreover, as the possibilities in question grade into each other, a dimensional analysis of consciousness as such can be effected, so that all experienced differences shall have place upon the continuum of possibilities so arrived at.

The fundamental variables of this system are described as those of *alliance* with its opposite *opposition*, and of *increase* with its opposite *decrease*, all expressing relations between stimulus and the ongoing activity of the organism. There are held to be four main possibilities, forming, as one might say, the primary qualities of all response, the "elementary unit responses": (1) The incoming activity may be in opposition to the activity already going on, and this opposition may result in an increase in the latter activity, as when a baby grasps a rod tighter to resist its being pulled away from him. (2) There may be such opposition, but with resulting decrease in the pre-existent activity. (3) The incoming activity may harmonize with the pre-existent, and the result may be an increase in the latter. (4) There may be such harmony, but with resulting decrease. The four types are termed "dominance," "compliance," "in-

---

[62] Marston, King, and Marston, *op. cit.*, chap. xiv.

ducement," and "submission." Of each type there are numerous degrees, and these can be diagrammed in circular fashion, with dominance and submission, compliance and inducement, opposite each other on the circle, and thus equivalent formally to the four primary qualities of color. And indeed the correspondence must, by the principles of the system, be more than formal. The colors are described in terms of the relations of dominance, etc., between the visual stimulus and the self-activity of the optical system. Thus blue is dominance of the former over the latter; yellow is submission; green is compliance; red, inducement. In applying these conceptions to sensory rather than emotional phenomena there is a reversal of direction in the relations which need not here be explained since it does not affect the basic idea of an identical pattern for all phases of experience. The remaining senses are held to be subject to the same mode of explanation.

The resemblance of this scheme to that of Pikler, in spite of striking differences (the chief of which is that Pikler alone seems to make use of directly observed characteristics of color), is unmistakable. It is clear that the standard system of inexplicable qualities, irreducibly different from motor aspects of mind, will have henceforth to reckon with radically heterodox alternatives. The significance of this lies in the fact that the orthodox view has no scientific merit save this, that though it led to endless squabbling about details, or even about semigeneral questions, such as the question of the complexity of non-primary qualities, it did represent the absence of clear-cut alternatives. Such alternatives now exist, and therewith vanishes the last excuse for resting content with the doctrine that sensations cannot be understood, or that there is nothing in them to understand. A new era in sensory theory has been opened.[63]

[63] F. G. Boring's recent and important book, *The Physical Dimensions of Consciousness* (1933), expresses a compromise between atomistic and dimensional views. It accepts the principle that psychical attributes are dimensions; but in treating the attribute or dimension of quality it divides it into subdimensions, such as the four primary colors, and regards the relations between these as merely that of combination, i.e., it adopts at this point the atom-molecule view. If I am not mistaken, this represents well

## SECTION 21. BEHAVIOR, GESTALT, AND AFFECTIVE CONTINUITY

The usual neglect of psychological writers even to discuss the only theory which can treat consciousness as an intelligible whole—the theory of it as a potential continuum of affective tones—has grounds which the following quotation, taken from one who is far from sharing the point of view of this book,[64] may help to make clear:

> The task of modern psychology . . . . consists primarily in a bare description of the data of individual experience exactly as they are presented, *without inference or hypothesis*. Although this task may seem direct and simple, it is in point of fact difficult of attainment and complex in its results. The reason for this *lies in the inveterate tendency of the physical and common-sense intellect to employ the immediate data of experience merely as symbols of something lying outside of that particular experience*. Even pleasure and pain are usually regarded in this light and in everyday life it is *only in aesthetic mood* that we appreciate the nature of color experiences in their own right.[65]

In this quotation the longer italicized passage states a cause almost sufficient of itself to explain the overlooking of the essential emotionalities of sensory contents. In addition, though unwittingly, the first italicized passage suggests a further cause. Charles Darwin said: "A good observer really means a good theorist," and "There can be no serviceable observation except for or against some theory." But if accuracy of observation is partially dependent upon accuracy of thought, and if all accuracy of thought depends, as I hold (sec. 26), upon the principle of continuity, then there is no reason to suppose that observation performed in essential conflict with that principle can

---

the present state of psychology, a state of transition between two schemes of analysis. The relation between subdimensions of quality which the facts suggest is that of intersection, e.g., at the point of mid-gray. It is true that Professor Boring has primarily the physiological dimensions in mind and assumes the three-process theory of vision. But in the end he will have to explain the phenomena as given, and these exhibit no mixtures of color qualities whatsoever, but only degrees and intersecting dimensions of likeness and difference. Would it not be as well to begin with an accurate analysis of these?

[64] Except that he is, or unfortunately, because of his untimely death since this was written, I must say was, a panpsychist.

[65] L. T. Troland, *The Present Status of Visual Science*, p. 15. Italics mine.

have any great value. Finally, the third italicized passage is a vivid though unintentional indication that the attitude of qualitative observation is basically aesthetic, and therefore that the presupposition, common to most psychologists, that the essential facts of sensation can be arrived at without the employment of aesthetic categories is fallacious.

Suppose a psychology aiming to describe "experience as such" is a feasible enterprise. Then the following remarks by a distinguished aesthetician point out a truth whose significance for this enterprise is manifest: "Art expresses experience simply as such."[66] "The condition of aesthetic experience is no more than the condition of being presented merely as an experience."[67] It follows that "all experience, in fact, is without exception aesthetic"[68] and that the aesthetic aspect of mind is "the most primitive and fundamental thing in conscious life." These words are not spoken idly, but upon the basis of abundant experience and keen analysis.

Does it follow that the method of psychology should be to lose ourselves in sheer aesthetic enjoyment? No, for the method of any science must be analytic, and that of psychology must be experimental as well. But it does follow that the categories brought to bear upon data must be in part aesthetic categories, and that we must rid ourselves of the prejudice that certain data are subjective because they are affective. Affective tones are subjective in precisely the sense that all the subject-matter of introspective psychology is so, namely, affective tones are the stuff of which immediate experience is made. We may study the space-time quantities of the physical world, or the logical relations of pure mathematics, without explicit mention of affective tones; but if the subject-matter of our study is subjectivity itself, then it is precisely these affective tones, despised of every other science, that we have to study as our objective facts. A psychologist writes:

[66] Lascelles Abercrombie, *Toward a Theory of Art*, p. 53.
[67] *Ibid.*, pp. 33-34.   [68] *Ibid.*, p. 26.

All experience is significant. Even its most trivial and evanescent phases have a certain objective reference and specific worth in our ideal syntheses. Throughout the whole web of experience runs the thread of this subjective valuation, giving significance and emotional quality to its stream.[69]

Yet this author holds that psychology itself cannot describe experience in this immediately significant, or qualitative, aspect, but only in terms of its causal uniformitites and physiological conditions. This, I suspect, is for psychology the real issue. Perhaps the problem of immediacy is too delicate for experimental investigation? But who shall say how far our methods might be refined?

The question may be discussed in relation to three prominent tendencies in recent psychology: behaviorism, Gestalt psychology, and psychoanalysis.

The first is an intelligible reaction against traditional introspective psychology, with its admission of mysterious ultimates and its inability to reach agreement concerning such "irreducible" elements or classes of phenomena. But, in its more extreme forms at least, it is unacceptable, for three main reasons. First, it maintains in effect that all knowable orders of things are capable of adequate arrangement in the four-dimensional manifold of physics. This is contrary to fact. The "direction" or order from red to green through yellow is not identical with any space-time direction whatsoever. The fact that the stimuli to these sensations form an order of space-time magnitudes does not entitle us to substitute this order for the manifestly different order of sensations.

In the second place, behaviorism is not acceptable in so far as it regards as of no consequence numerous researches, such as that which we have reviewed upon the "characters" of *sensa*, whose value is apparent. For although this work remains, as introspectionists have treated it, highly unsatisfactory, it nevertheless establishes the existence of introspective psychology as a genuine science. Such researches accomplish the one absolute essential of science: They force general ideas to come into more intimate and detailed contact than would otherwise have oc-

---

[69] Robert MacDougall, *General Problems of Psychology*, p. 334.

curred with facts observable by a technique repeatable by other investigators, and applied in a spirit of unexceptionable scientific fairness. They elicit with clearness facts whose existence might have remained only vaguely suspected. They invite further speculation upon an already established and not hopelessly inadequate factual basis. Our gratitude for such researches should be immense, and we cannot for a moment adopt the attitude of arrogant wholesale detraction that is characteristic of behaviorism.

In the third place, in order to maintain the profound truth, that mind and behavior are all of one piece, we do not need to admit that mind is nothing but the translation of dead matter through space. We need rather to discover in mind as its essential trait an organically active character, and to see in the body the social co-ordination of the lives of living cells constituted out of a similar activity. Introspection has made two paradoxically opposite errors: it has failed to describe immediacy fully in its own terms (what is the doctrine of modes but a hasty inference from physiology?); and, on the other hand, it has greatly exaggerated the gulf between mind and body. Provided that the body be seen as genuinely alive in all its parts—a life which seen from without is cell behavior; from within, individual integrations or centers of feeling constituting the cells as they are in themselves—the mind of the human individual may then be defined as this bodily life focused in a single immediacy of aesthetic value;[70] and the observation of facts immediately included in this focus may be greatly aided by this conception. In short, it is only the negations of behaviorism that we need negate. As for the scientific observability of immediacy, this depends perhaps above all upon the judicious use—as yet almost untried—of geometrical analysis, providing an impersonally precise frame of reference for questions and answers. And if immediacy is intrinsically active and fused with the life of the bodily cells, then an "inner" state has also always an outer aspect, so that public or behavioristic observation is in principle

[70] Cf. Whitehead, *Science and the Modern World*, p. 128.

always relevant to "private" states.[71] Pragmatism is the essential truth of behaviorism; purpose is the Janus-like inner-outer by which both mind and matter are made intelligible. For purpose is felt tendency to act, a "content" or mental state which is given as actually or potentially on its way to action. Analysis can, upon this basis, be applied to both the "ineffable" contents of consciousness and the concept of consciousness itself.

Gestalt psychology is in a general way favorable to an affective and geometrical theory of mind. But it seems as yet too little perceived that the organic conception of immediacy can in one aspect be accurately expressed only through the notion of a continuum, and in another only through an affective conception of mind. How closely Gestalt psychology can approach to the concept of affective continuity may be seen in a recent book on the subject.[72] It should more and more be realized that it is folly to oppose materialistic behaviorism with a program which repeats that abstraction from the subtler conceptions of value which is precisely the gist of such behaviorism. The behaviorist understands business values and engineering values, and mind in this sense, well enough. Mind as a pattern of enjoyment nuances is the essential thing that he neglects. In Gestalt psychology this defect is not wholly overcome.[73]

As for psychoanalysis, its methodological implication seems to be that nothing is to be taken more seriously, in any study of mind, than the aspect of desire and valuation. Psychoanalysis tends to discredit utterly the old idea of mind as primarily cognitive, in the sense of barely registrative of reality, without essential reference to valuation, and to discredit also the idea of consciousness as first of all private and only secondarily other-regarding. The seeming absence of the consciousness of values in theoretical work ought henceforth to be interpreted as indi-

[71] How far we are from the carrying-out of this program is shown by the failure thus far of all attempts to establish response correlates for pleasantness and unpleasantness (see Beebe-Center, *op. cit.*, chaps. viii and ix).

[72] Köhler, *op. cit.*, pp. 240–64.

[73] This is the principal criticism brought against the movement in the most elaborate critical study yet devoted to it (see Martin Scheerer, *Die Lehre von der Gestalt* [Berlin and Leipzig, 1931], pp. 143, 144 n., 278–79).

cating the automatic sway of valuations which have dropped below the level of clear consciousness, partly through their habitual character, partly because their recognition is "censored" by the conventions of science. Psychoanalytic experience further indicates that the way to bring into clearer consciousness these hidden springs of mental action is to take seriously every variety of dream utterance, in particular that great variety called "art." It is the artists whose business it is to give away the secrets of the soul, in despite of all "censors." It is they above all who wish to intuit life in its totality and as it is, for it is they alone who, in any full sense, place life higher than conventional abstractions; they alone who seek to make explicit what man inwardly and essentially is. In spite of such suggestions no such thing as a general method for psychology conceived as a science can be extracted from Freud or his followers.

It is generally recognized that the rise of psychology as a science is due to the stimulating example of modern physics. Yet there is one consequence of this which is perhaps not so frequently realized. The history of physics shows clearly enough that the successful scientific method consists in the refinement, by mathematical and experimental means, of certain instinctive or common-sense beliefs derived from everyday life. Now modern psychology arose when the intellectual world was preoccupied with physics as an already well-accredited science. Instead, therefore, of seeking an independent source for itself in primordial human intuitions, comparable to the intuition of the physical environment as capable of mechanical control upon which physics had been founded, psychology regarded common sense as discredited pre-science, and sought to found itself directly upon the model of physics. Since this model was too remotely analogous to suffice, the resort was had, not to really basic intuition, but to such more or less outworn philosophy as is always ingrained in the modes of thought fashionable among educated men of any given age. Intellectual fashions and (now antiquated) physics, not the knowledge of the mind which all men have simply as men, became the foundation. Now the fact is that there is a large region of such really primordial knowledge which is of no direct relevance to physics (except via physiology) but is decidedly pertinent to psychology, and which is a more reliable clue to the nature of mind than the supposed analogy of the parts or elements of consciousness to the atoms of physics or the elements of chemistry.[74] This knowledge is primarily concerned with the emotional tones pervading all experience and unifying all its phases and species.

Contemporary psychology shows a conflict of prejudices which there is no ground for supposing can be overcome except in some such way as the following. Observation must be in connection with specific well-considered hypotheses. These must be formulated in terms, on the one hand, of continuity and its geometrical and quantitative aspects; in terms, on the other, of value, aesthetic affection, and social relationships. Traditional psychology has dwelt in a sort of vacuum between the intelligibility and accuracy of scientific concepts, on the one side, and the more elusive but fundamental implications of practical, aesthetic, and social experiences, on the other.

There is but one way out of the present impasse—a genuine and deliberate synthesis of these two eternally valid points of view. This synthesis must be at the price of the abandonment of much of that semi-science of introspective psychology whose half-successes constitute the chief enigma and yet perhaps the chief promise of contemporary thought.

[74] See subsecs. 6A, B, C, E.

# CHAPTER V

# DUALISM IN AESTHETICS

**\*\***

*This immediately interested, wholly self-reliant experience which we call aesthetic .... may occur wherever intuition is vivid enough to provide its own valuation.*

*A face-value .... that does not call for reference to anything outside itself.*

LASCELLES ABERCROMBIE

**\*\***

### SECTION 22. THE PREMISSES OF AESTHETICS

THREE facts in aesthetic theory are not in dispute. The first is that an aesthetically enjoyable object is given as coherent, as bound together into a more closely unified perceptual whole than are non-aesthetic objects. The only qualification is that this unity must not be so rigid as to exclude variety or create monotony. To take this condition into account we may employ the phrase "coherent diversity." The second indisputable fact is that the aesthetically enjoyed object is, at least in the most pronounced cases, the object of intensely concentrated and absorbed attention. If it is a visual object, it is intensely seen; if auditory, it is vividly heard. The third indisputable fact is that the aesthetically enjoyed object is enjoyed—that, accordingly, aesthetic experience involves feeling. It is in reference to these three recognized features that controversial questions ought to be considered. Our question becomes, in simplest terms, this: Can aesthetic enjoyments be explained or described in terms simply of the absorbed contemplation of coherent perceptual patterns of color or sound? By Occam's razor, we should refrain from the introduction of further factors until their necessity be shown.

The principle of coherent diversity comprises two main features. The first of these is the similarity of the parts to one another, not only with respect to their simple qualities of color or sound, but also with respect to the arrangement of these in space and time. Everywhere, in all artistic objects whatsoever, inspection discloses more extensive likenesses between the parts than occur in non-aesthetic objects other than those whose aesthetic nullity is clearly due to an excess of likeness, of uniformity. These repetitions of theme, of motif, with more or less variation are completely universal characters of art. In a painting they may be far from obvious, but careful examination discloses their presence to an extent explicable only by the supposition that the aesthetic feeling required them. If there are in a picture a house, a tree, and a cloud, there will be more than a chance degree of similarity in the outlines of these objects, either among themselves or in relation to other objects in the picture. It is in this way that "distortions" of nature inevitably arise. The second main feature of the principle of coherence is the interpenetration of the parts of the aesthetic whole in the sense that the perception of each includes the perception of all.[1] However one may seek to limit the focus of attention upon, for example, a single color in a picture, the surrounding colors remain included, at least in the "fringe" of this act of attention, so that the separate colors are never seen purely in themselves but always as differing from, contrasted with, or akin to, neighboring colors. There is no psychological reality corresponding to the idea of color except as a contrast effect, as a term in a relation of likeness or difference to other colors. As one shifts attention from part to part of the picture one does not apprehend it as items $x+y+z$, but as $x(y, z)+y(x, z)+z(x, y)$, the factors in parentheses representing elements in the fringe of attention. Only in this sense is the picture a composite of parts.[2] It will be

---

[1] This is only partially true in the "time arts," such as music, since the future is not, except in a general way, given in the present (in spite of the well-known assertion of Mozart, who can hardly have intended to assert an absolute suppression of time in his creative visions).

[2] "In the moment of aesthetic enjoyment there are not parts seen or rather thought in their relations. The relations denoted by balance, harmony, .... form, are relations apprehended in immediacy, i.e., such that both the relations and the relata are all one quality" (Philip Leon; see Carritt, *Philosophies of Art*, p. 287).

observed that interpenetration is a matter of degree, in that the extent to which neighboring parts suffer the vagueness or faintness inherent in the fringe or extra-focal part of attention varies endlessly.

The necessity of interpenetration furnishes the key to the necessity of similarity. For interpenetration, integration, of perceptions implies their partial identity, and the partially identical is in so far the not wholly dissimilar. And in fact where similarity of quality or form is relatively lacking, the attempt to embrace the parts in a single unity of attention will also achieve but relative success. There will be a sense of confusion, or of rivalry between the parts, such that either none will be perceived with distinctness, or else the clear perception of any one will be attained only at the price of almost complete obscurity for the others.

The law of aesthetic order is then the twofold but inseparably unitary one of coherence as uniformity and coherence as mutual internality. The uniformity is, however, blended with the exceptional, the law-abiding with the irregular, necessity with freedom (in music and the temporal arts, anticipation with surprise); and the mutual inclusion admits of degrees of vividness. Just as particles pervade, through their "fields" of energy, from which they cannot be conceived abstracted, all other particles, but are more and more faintly operative in each other the greater the distance between them, so the influence of colors upon each other is diminished with distance apart in the picture. Hence, in both cases, the illusion of complete externality, absolute independence.

Such is the order of the aesthetic object. Whence, then, is the enjoyment—not to mention the depth of significance and "expressiveness"—which we derive from this object? Is it self-evident that coherent and hence relatively clear perceptions should issue in enjoyment? The following considerations force us to confess that an understanding of the aesthetic response ("that is beautiful," "that is artistic") presupposes a principle which we have not yet made explicit, a principle as old as Greek philosophy and at present the predominant concept in aesthetic discussion the world over. We refer to the principle of "expression," of the "embodiment," in the sensory object, of emotions and feelings, conceived as states distinct from mere sense perceptions or mere ratiocinations.

1. In the first place, even the most simple and isolated colors, tones, and odors can have an appeal in no way adequately explained by structure. And, although coherence of structure does guarantee vividness, facility, and amplitude of perception, nevertheless it is fully as plausible to explain the value of structural unity in terms of the values of the individual tones or colors as to reverse the process. When the parts of an aesthetic object harmonize, this means that they reinforce each other in their individual effects instead of tending to interfere with each other or cancel each other out. But if each in itself has no value proper to itself, no contribution of its own to make, it cannot matter whether or not these nonexistent contributions conflict or agree. Thus a harmonious society is valuable because in it each individual is enabled to be something individually significant, is enabled to be more completely himself than he could be in a condition of social chaos. It has been remarked that a harmony of psychological impulses is valuable because it means a more complete realization of the potentialities of the organism, and because "it is better to be fully than partially alive."[3] But this is precisely the assertion that every fragment of experience has its intrinsic value, as a fragment of experience, as a bit of being alive. And this is just what the intellectualists in aesthetics have been gratuitously seeking to avoid by the hypothesis that all the value lies in the structural element alone, while the sensuous simple qualities are, in the sense in which life is better than death, not alive at all![4]

From the concepts of order and of the mere capacity to cognize that order there is no evident path to the concepts of feeling, of joy and sorrow, of love and hate. Even that the intuition

---

[3] C. K. Ogden, I. A. Richards, and James Wood, *Foundations of Aesthetics*, p. 91.

[4] From this point of view, the Crocean doctrine of the "identity" of intuition and expression, which for the authors of the *Foundations of Aesthetics* is an empty phrase, is simply the immediate or qualitative aspect of the doctrine expounded in that book!

of order is pleasing to us is intelligible only if we suppose that the intuition involves a kernel of desiring or valuing, i.e., that this intuition is not "merely cognitive," a pure registration of facts, but is also a mode of feeling, in so far as it cares about the degree of its own success or failure. But in that case, why pretend that mere order and order registration are the decisive categories? Obviously, feeling is the implied clue to the whole matter. After all, feeling might conceivably generate order, whereas order by itself can in valid logic generate only order.

2. If the immediate realization of value is that which ought to be called "feeling," then the intrinsic value of aesthetic experience is wholly due to its affective character. But the aesthetic experience is intensely perceptual, and is unusually free from distractions from the objects as given. Granting these factors of an exceptional objectivity of attention and an exceptional enjoyment of feeling, we have, as a result, that the condition of the feeling, the absorption in the object, seems to require that the feeling be as little attended to as possible, lest it distract from the object; although the feeling, since it is the intrinsic worth of the experience, should be as vividly experienced as possible. This requirement seems to amount to saying that the feeling and the object should be included in a focus of attention maximal for both. We have seen that the condition of inclusion in a single act of attention, which is interpenetration in the Bergsonian sense, is a sufficient degree of similarity of the elements to be attended to. It seems to follow that the sensory pattern which yields the value feeling must be like it, or the two will compete as to which is to be relegated to the dulness of the psychic fringe. Neither can in fact be sacrificed; neither in fact is sacrificed.

3. The principle of coherence itself is applicable universally to sense data only if we concede their essentially affective character. Red and green, orange and blue, "cohere" aesthetically. This means that they form a stable integration, allowing co-contribution to a single focus of maximal attention. Integration means partial identity, hence similarity. In any case, the explanation of coherence through partial similarity is so generally

applicable that we should not abandon the principle at any point without careful inquiry. We must consider the hypothesis that even colors so widely separated as to be complementary are yet in some sense exceptionally similar. As we have seen in an earlier discussion (sec. 5C), conventional psychology is quite inconsistent in its account of the similarities of color qualities. Can it furnish us with the similarities required to explain harmony?

An authority on the aesthetics of color, Mr. Denman Ross, answers in the affirmative. He states his position as follows:

> Whenever two or more impressions or ideas have something in common that is appreciable, they are in harmony.....[5]
> 
> By tone-harmony I mean a relation of likeness in tones.....[6]
> 
> Tone-harmony resolves itself into Value-harmony, Color-harmony [usually called "analogous harmony"], harmony between hues or shades of some one color, such as red, and the Harmony of Intensities [meaning by intensity degree of *saturation*].[7]

What this means is that harmony between non-analogous colors, such as scarlet and green, would have to be regarded—and Mr. Ross so regards it—as due entirely to likenesses of value (brightness) or of saturation. Yet yellow and purple are surely more harmonious—other things being equal—than yellow and orange, although they have less resemblance on one of Mr. Ross's possible dimensions of harmony (the dimension of value), no more on a second (saturation), and less—indeed, so far as his account goes, none at all—on a third ("color"). It seems fair to conclude that Mr. Ross has here relied too much upon conventional psychology. His "color"-harmony is obviously two-dimensional, so that yellow and purple must, in one respect, be at least as much alike as yellow and orange are in two respects. Moreover, since it is in aesthetic experience that the intuition of qualitative unity becomes prominent, why should we not expect such experience to reveal also the nature of this unity, the respects of similarity so intuited? Now aesthetic phenomena do in fact afford suggestions concerning the variables of which complementary

[5] *The Theory of Pure Design* (New York: Houghton, Mifflin and Company, 1917), p. 1.
[6] *Ibid.*, p. 158.
[7] *Ibid.* The same theory was held by Ostwald.

colors are at once opposed and yet approximately equal values. Red is felt in artistic appreciation as warm, insistent, advancing; its bluish-green complementary is cool, gentle, receding. Yellow is lively, cheerful, light-hearted; blue-violet is quiet, wistful, earnest. But in the respect in which one pair of complementaries are opposed, the other is not opposed; thus yellow and violet agree in that neither is so warm as red nor so cool as green; red and green in that both are serious rather than gay, like yellow, or sad, like violet. Thus complementation means at once strong contrast and close likeness. This fulfils both the aesthetic requirement of unity in variety and the inexorable logical requirement of a two-dimensional circular system, such as the colors, apart from brightness, constitute. Those who believe that such terms as "warmth" or "gaiety" really describe (admittedly crudely) not the color qualities themselves, but only associative accretions of the colors, have on their side the burden of proof that the aesthetic and logical requirements can upon the associative assumption be met.

It is not necessary for the argument that exact complementaries should have preference, for the extreme contrast in one dimension may be felt as somewhat violent in spite of the affinity in the other dimension. It may be felt as a smoother harmony if a less complete identity along one variable makes possible a less violent contrast along the other, as in yellow and purple, or red and yellow-green. Experiment supports this view.[8] The least harmonious pairs, on the other hand, will clearly be those which have in both dimensions the maximum contrasts which are simultaneously possible, as in scarlet and yellow, each of which is a midvalue of that which the other represents in its extreme; and the most violently discordant pairs will be those which are close enough on both dimensions strongly to suggest, yet far enough definitely to inhibit, the sense that they are but variations of the same color. Thus, starting with any point of the color circle, there will be a small section of the circle around this point which will include the colors in "analo-

---

[8] See J. G. Beebe-Center, *Pleasantness and Unpleasantness*, p. 133. For results apparently inconsistent with these see Marion Ofner's Master's Thesis, *The Affective Value of Color Combinations*, The University of Chicago.

gous harmony" with it, those that are but slight modifications of the "same" color. Beyond both ends of this section there will be two sections of positive conflict shading into relative unrelatedness, then the entire remainder of the circle, which will involve in both directions a transition from relative unrelatedness along both to relatedness along one dimension, but with increasing distance along the other, and this may finally overcome part of the advantage of the one-dimensional approach, so that there may be two maxima of complementary harmony in this section, separated by a somewhat less harmonious region of full complementarism. (For a diagram of color relations see p. 222.)

This explanation of the main facts of color-harmony depends upon the reality of the Cartesian co-ordinates which non-affective theories of sensation leave in obscurity or deny altogether. It is in favor of the principles upon which the explanation is based that they also apply to the problem of musical harmony. The ability to recognize the place of a note within its octave more easily than the octave itself is so violent a paradox that the theory of "octave quality" has been devised to explain it, together with the facts of fusion. But the remaining intervals and their degrees of harmony and discord can also be explained in a similar manner, although this seems not to have been noticed.[9] Namely, if octave quality, like color quality apart from brightness, is two-dimensional, then the pure tones ascend not in a straight line like the grays but in a spring-shaped spiral; and if we abstract from pitch and consider octave quality alone, we must see this as a circle upon which the relationships are analogous to those of the saturated colors. Notes an octave apart coincide upon the circle; hence their tendency to fuse. Major thirds are exactly one-third of the way around the circle from each other, or two-thirds of halfway—in short, are two-thirds of the distance which would render them "complementaries" in the color sense. Now colors so separated are, other things being equal, maximally harmonious. Again, minor thirds are half-complementaries, a slightly inharmonious interval. Notes a whole tone apart are one-third complementaries — a separation

[9] On the usual explanations of musical harmony see sec. 33.

which is about the worst of the color intervals and is also decidedly the least concordant of sound relationships. Halftones are one-sixth complementaries, like scarlet and orange, that is to say, not far from analogous harmony, yet still removed from it. And so they seem to me to sound. Notes eight halftones apart are two-thirds complementary, reckoning the opposite way around the circle; but this relationship is not found in colors when they are saturated, since saturated colors reach their maximal brightness separation at the complementary interval (blue and yellow), whereas tones continue to increase in pitch interval all the way through the octave. Thus augmented fifths are less closely related than thirds in pitch while equally so in octave quality; whereas red is equidistant both in hue and in brightness from yellow-green and green-blue. Augmented fifths are related as are red and green-blue mixed with considerable white. As this implies, the harmony is not marked. The octave relationship itself is like that of red and pink, relatively harmless and relatively unexciting. With tuning forks octaves are insipid, all too similar, while major thirds are irresistible, sweet yet strong, like near but not too near complementaries—deep scarlet and yellow-green. The other tone relationships are also at least roughly as the color analogy would imply. Now the moral is that the explanation of color-harmony in terms of similarities occult to ordinary psychology but at least vaguely definable in terms of an affective theory of the dimensions of sensory quality (the "warmth" common to orange and purple, e.g.) may perhaps apply also to harmony of sounds, and in both cases seems to be the only explanation that can admit a unitary principle underlying all harmony. The feeling of harmony is intelligible if and only if the elements which it relates are themselves of the nature of feeling.

4. We have seen that mere coherence of elements not in themselves affective cannot explain satisfaction as a feeling. On the other hand, from the assumption of the essential emotionality of the sensory elements, coherence follows as an obvious correlate. For of course emotional tones should cohere, since this means only that they should permit each other to exist without

loss of vividness, without mutual destruction; and if emotions are intrinsically good, the more of them the better, so long as their number does not involve proportionate loss in the vividness of each.

That one exceptionally vivid feeling all by itself cannot equal a harmonious plurality is an obvious inference from the structure of existence itself. So long, for instance, as there is memory of past feeling, the present cannot be free from emotional complexity. The only question is as to the harmony of this complexity. All the grounds for the complexity itself are perhaps summed up in the statement that the essence of existence is social, that being itself is a social transaction. A harmony of emotions is a society in its simplest terms; for an emotional disharmony is a disturbance which presupposes the coherence which it disrupts.

The conclusion from the foregoing is that, so far as they function in aesthetic experience at all, sense data are scarcely distinguishable from emotional tones. This follows from the whole natural spirit of aesthetic affirmation, which is objective and enjoying in one, a feeling which is perception, a perception which is feeling. Either the feeling must be transparent, and hence not vivid or distinctive in itself, so that the object may appear clearly through it, or, if the feeling is to be fully realized in its distinctive character, it must coincide with the object which equally is to be realized. The absorption of attention in the object is then conceived as identically absorption in an intrinsic value as such. We love and behold things either for themselves, and as ends, or else as means and instruments. But nothing is more than an instrument save living feeling and emotion. The attempt to interpret the aesthetic datum as at once intrinsically beloved and yet (as given) not intrinsically alive and emotional—that is to say, genuinely lovable—is the fundamental contradiction of modern aesthetics. There is but one love, the participation of life in life, of feeling in feeling. The rest is either a faint degree of this or the mere utilization of a tool which, as such, is not even so much as regarded or beheld consciously at all. To behold it we must abandon the attitude of mere use and adopt that of aesthetic fusion of the object with an objectified feeling.

### SECTION 23. EXPRESSION AND ASSOCIATION

The doctrine of expressionism is in its strictest form neatly summed up in the often gibed at, often admired, and sometimes understood, Crocean formula: art = intuition (immediate knowledge) = expression. This doctrine admits of the following forms, according as the relation between the feeling "embodied" and the sense data which embody it is interpreted.

There is first a broad distinction between doctrines which rely entirely upon the principle of association as the ground of expression, and those which posit some other mode of connection. The word "association" is here used to mean any doctrine which ascribes the entire feeling import of a sense content to the fact that feeling and content happen to occur together in experience, rather than to a relatedness logically inherent in the natures of sensation and feeling. In short, the contrast is between merely existential and essential connectedness.

Among associational doctrines we may distinguish "tight" and "loose" forms, according to the strength, permanence, and universality of the association linkages. The extreme of looseness is found in the view that the feeling values depend upon purely personal and more or less radically alterable associations —as that a certain color might seem joyous because of some flowers of that color which recently had been received under happy circumstances. Should one's feelings toward the sender subsequently fade or undergo unfortunate reversal, the meaning of the color might then also change radically. The extreme of tightness is the hypothesis that the connections are innate to the race, and perhaps to the higher animals. There must then doubtless be an inborn connection between the nerve processes underlying the feelings and those underlying the sensations.

The extreme loose doctrine reduces art creation to a pure gamble. How could the artist know the effect which his colors or sounds would have if this effect depended for each person upon the most accidental and unique aspects of his personal history?

Philosophers may assert this doctrine; but they should know that they are making nonsense of art. And it is certainly not the fact that artists interpret their task in this light.[10] What artist ever put himself on record as so believing? A less frivolous doctrine would be that the decisive aesthetic associations were mainly determined by social conventions and thus might vary from age to age or from culture to culture but would present considerable uniformities within any one culture. Thus Occidentals may share in certain color feelings or sound feelings which to Orientals are quite or largely foreign, and thus what are discords to one age or people may be agreeable tone combinations to another. Against this doctrine are the following facts: in the case of colors, at least, no striking evidences of such cultural differences have been found; where the use of colors is different, the simplest explanation, fitting all the facts, is not that the same colors express different feelings to different peoples, but that different peoples, having different feelings to express, have embodied this difference of feeling in a difference of color. For example, the often quoted use of white (and indeed of many other colors) in funerals by the Chinese (and for that matter by many other peoples) is no proof whatsoever that the Chinese feeling for white is different from ours (do we not call white a "pure" color, see in it a certain detachment from the passions and the joys of life?) but suggests rather that the Chinese do not share our conviction that the symbols connected with a funeral should be such as to express solely the sheer negativity, destructiveness, and despair of death, which our black does for us (and would, I believe, also do for the Chinese). The fact is that white expresses here not evil but sacredness; the Chinese put the religious meaning first, as many have held we should do.[11]

Again, if a savage prefers somewhat cruder colors than the rest of us, so are the feelings which they express for him (and for

---

[10] See the important book by Ozenfant, himself a painter: *Foundations of Modern Art* (New York: Brewer, Warren & Putnam, 1931), chaps. x and xi.

[11] The funeral ceremonies of any ancestor-worshipping people are partly designed to placate or serve the spirits of the departed. The Chinese carry effigies, such as paper automobiles, to be burned and thus sent to the departed. Not only white but red and other colors are used. Clearly there is no intention of furnishing the emotional equiva-

us) more crude than the feelings we may wish to enjoy. I repeat that there is no evidence that culture determines color feeling, but only that it affects color preference or evaluation, a very different thing. It is one thing to find the play a sad one; it is quite another to like or not to like it, to prefer or not to prefer it to a gay one.

Similar remarks apply to musical discords. There is no reason to suppose that the coming into vogue of a certain combination of sounds previously condemned as inharmonious means that the feeling tone of this combination becomes something quite new. There is the other possibility, namely, that a feeling tone previously disliked comes now, in a more robust, less saccharine and conventionalized age, to be appreciated for its very painfulness, its slight spice of tragedy. Precisely such changes in attitude toward feelings do occur. Nor, again, is there any reason to suppose that the nasal chanting in Chinese theaters is enjoyed because to the audience it conveys the quintessence of meltingly sweet sentiment, such as we seem to require. "Sweet" intonations are used on occasion, but it appears on the whole that the Chinese appreciate other feelings,[12] with a more mildly sweet character about them (for they are not to us wholly harsh) than some of our sentimentalists do. The instruments used with the action have a spicy, dramatic character, an emotional tenseness and piquancy, which one need only attend to, to feel; and doubtless many who have said that "the acting was wonderful but the music was too much for me," did not know

---

lent of our own ghastly, spiritless ceremony. The origin of black clothes seems to have been an intention to warn of the uncleanness of those having to do with a corpse rather than to indicate mourning. Black is a perfect sense symbol of death, but a less perfect one of grief.

[12] Ozenfant, however, says: "There are some people who question the universality of art. They say: 'Chinese music means little to us.' But does jazz mean nothing to the Chinese? It moves them despite their conventions. . . . . Chinese music is super-refined, but for the Chinese themselves, is it, after all, any more than a lulling caress? . . . . "The 'Pastoral Symphony' might seem gross to a refined Manchu, for the very reason that the decadent of today prefers a 'modern' figurine to some magnificent Easter Island idol, and a complicated musical trifle to the impressive tom-toms of Thibet. But it is Easter Island that prevails against Monet, Beethoven against the Chinese, Goethe against Mallarmé, the Thibetans against the Conservatoire of Music" (*op. cit.*, pp. 309-10).

that in fact the music conveyed its message to them at many a moment when they forgot to think about it or to indulge in mistaken theorizing about the purpose of art, which is to convey a feeling to you, to a certain extent whether you like the feeling or not.[13]

But the objections to the cultural theory go still deeper. There are at least two groups of facts which tempt us to conceive of certain important aesthetic associations as common to the human race, and even, in some cases, to the higher animals. On the one hand, there is scarcely any doubt but that such connections as light with goodness, darkness with evil, or such sounds as the growl or snarl with a hostile intention, are experienced at least by all humankind if not also by the higher animals. On the other hand, the causes which would tend to bring about such a uniformity are no utter mystery. All day-living animals at least must feel the directly beneficent character of sunlight, in which they may be seen to bask so luxuriously. But more than this, such classifications as warm colors, joyous colors, etc., as are to be found in almost any manual for workers in the visual arts correspond closely to a pattern of associations rooted in the biological past of the race. To take one example only, the warm, aggressive, insistent character of red can be ascribed to the fact that it is the color of blood, the only important, pervasively present red object in nature, and an object of the highest and most immediate concern in many ways. All the great

---

[13] There is also the well-known argument that, whereas in Europe the minor scale is regarded as sad, many peoples have songs written in this scale which to them are joyous. But this of course is not a difference of aesthetic experience but of (highly careless) aesthetic theorizing. Nobody can, except in a very special sense, experience "the minor key," which is not a sensory quality or any particular pattern of such qualities, but rather a highly complicated and abstract system of such patterns. To be sure, on the affective theory, the difference between the two systems must be an emotional difference, but this could not possibly be so elementary and direct a contrast as that of joy—sorrow, which must be capable of some degree of expression in any such system. It is as though, because the Euclidean and non-Euclidean geometries differ in structure, we were to infer that the one must be devoted exclusively to straight lines and angles and the other to curves and their intersections. The minor-key sadness, major-key gladness theorists are the aesthetic equivalents of those lay physicists whose knowledge of Einstein is exhausted in familiarity with the phrase "curved space." As for real experience, surely anyone can be made to sense happiness and sadness by music in any key through the appropriate melodic and tonal devices permitted in each. No difference in experience between persons or groups has here been demonstrated.

color meanings lend themselves to such explanations; and the correlations are too exact to leave much likelihood that these interpretations are purely fanciful.[14] Sounds present a more complicated problem, but here too there is universality with a natural biological basis.[15] It is upon such elemental "associations," if they are truly that, that the artist relies, not upon the trivial idiosyncrasies of personal history, nor even upon those of national history. The reasonableness of the artistic enterprise appears thus to be proportional to the power of these elemental linkages to hold their own in spite of all personal factors.

If we seek a more thorough analysis of the nature of the associations in question, we find three possibilities. First, the connections may not be inherited but may be developed anew in each individual. The uniformity of result, so far as it exists, would be due to the uniformity of environmental factors. Everyone sees much of the sky, most men see a good deal at least of foliage and of blood. And besides, these things enter into the tradition, so that the influence of literature and language and artistic usage would tend to extend their effects even, for example, upon a child of the city streets. And yet this account is not wholly satisfactory. It would imply, after all, rather drastic differences between city dwellers and country folk, between those living in regions where snow is common and those who have never seen snow (with clouds, the chief experience of white in nature); moreover, it would be strange if personal and eccentric associations should not frequently exert a decisive influence. Many will allege that precisely such variations occur. I am content here to urge that while the evidence is somewhat uncertain, it is clear that it would be an advantage to the artist if such variations were not to be feared, and that it is also doubtful whether any artist works with the possibility of them in mind.

Let us therefore consider the remaining possibilities of explanation. These are two views of innate associations. According to one of these, the mechanism which produces the sensations in question is innately integrated with a mechanism which

---

[14] See sec. 38A.     [15] See sec. 38B.

produces the feelings. I shall call this the dualistic form of innate associations. This doctrine is open to many objections of a serious kind. There is the general fact that such innate integrations appear rather exceptional in the makeup of the human mind, which is characterized by a remarkable freedom in its responses from any such predetermined patterns. Consider, for example, the discovery that all but two or three causes of fear are such because of individual experience or learning, and that this is true even of the higher animals as well as of human beings. Yet, since one of these innately fearful sensations is a loud sound, and since this fact is obviously relevant to the question of musical expression, the possibility of innate associations as the basis of expression may be taken seriously. In a later chapter, however, we shall consider a form of association which admits innateness while yet demanding nothing further of the biologist than just the unquestioned innateness of the sensory response itself.[16]

Our present task, however, is to point out a difficulty inherent in all forms of associations (except that form above referred to which identifies the associative and the sensory response) and which I hold to be decisive against all of them. This is the fact that aesthetic experience directly reveals a more intimate connection between sense quality and feeling tone than that of mere togetherness, even inherited. For example, to glow with pleasure at the sight of a house with which we have agreeable associations is not identical with finding it aesthetically satisfactory. Nothing is more perfectly possible than to perceive clearly in such a case the aesthetically mediocre character of the object. And does anyone suppose that sufficiently happy associations would transform the harsh grindings and groanings of street cars into sublime music, or the sight of an average brick pile into a design to be compared with a fine oriental rug? Something further besides mere emotional associations is required. This something further is the factor of objectification; the feelings are not given merely as connected with the sensations, but as seeming to inhere in them, appearing to be "spread out upon

[16] See sec. 38.

the object." Thus the associational theory is forced to take on a more unambiguously expressionist tinge. The transition is seen clearly in Santayana's famous definition of beauty as "objectified pleasure." This objectification of the feeling into or upon the object as datum is more than even the tightest bond whereby the occurrence of the one element in consciousness entails the occurrence of the other. In addition to association, in short, we have fusion, the (actual or illusory) immanence of the feeling in the sense datum.

### SECTION 24. EXPRESSION AND IMMANENCE

Immanence appears to be open to four principal interpretations. The first may be called the confusion theory; the second, the theory of inherence; the third, the similarity theory; the fourth, the identity theory.

The confusion theory is a hypothesis of illusion. A tonality is not really given as inhering in the sensum, but there is an illusion of its being so given. It is this illusion only which is directly apprehended. The feeling does not, in short, actually appear where the color or sound does, but only appears to appear there. The appeal of this theory is peculiarly strong to what have been well characterized as "obstinately verbal minds." Verbally we can describe a thing as hateful or odious without at all meaning that we directly perceive the feelings of hate or odium in the things. Similarly, it is thought, when an aesthetic subject reports that he sees the flowers as gay, the cloud as gloomy, he does not literally intuit such feelings as out there in space but only, by a confusion, imagines he so intuits them. The following is a peculiarly subtle expression of this hypothesis:

> While I do not deny that association plays a part in determining the *Stimmung* of colors, I believe that the direct effect of the stimulus upon the body plays a greater part. The light stimulus not only affects the sensory apparatus of the brain, where it causes a sensation of color, but overflows into muscular and glandular paths, producing some slight deviation from equilibrium there, the conscious aspect of which is a feeling.[17] Being diffuse and vague,

---

[17] Subjective feelings are the conscious aspects of muscular and glandular activities; but is there any evidence that objective feelings, those which alone are here in question, are of this character? It would be strange if the sense of good and evil, of desire, satis-

and not being connected with any conscious wish, this feeling seems not so much to be one's own, as to belong to the stimulus upon which it is suffused.[18]

We find here, in combination, the doctrine of mere sensation as something in itself not at all affective and the recognition of a feeling occurring simultaneously with the sensation and agreeing with it in the character of apparent objectivity ("seems not to be one's own . . . . suffused upon the stimulus"). The possibility of this objectification of the feeling upon an object already fully determinate in quality by virtue of the sensation alone is grounded in the diffuseness and vagueness of the former. I cannot refrain from suggesting that the vagueness is rather in the theory here expounded than in the feelings in question. For if the latter are so vague that they can without any perception of discrepancy be intuited as qualifying the sensory object, although the latter is simultaneously given as perfectly definite in its qualities of color or sound, so that there is no point at which such vague auras could appropriately be imagined to apply, then it is hard to see how such qualitative elasticities could impart to aesthetic feeling the subtle determinateness which it appears nevertheless to have. Moreover, it is not clear how even the most excessive vagueness could explain the confusion. I may, to be sure, think that an object in a fog is a man, a lamp post, or what not. But then it is with these objects as they would appear if indistinctly discerned that I confuse what I see. In aesthetic vision or audition, on the other hand, I have an unusually distinct perception of the sensory object as such. If in the qualities of this object as a datum nothing affective inheres, I am in a poor condition to undergo the illusion that the opposite is the case.

The second or attribute theory posits genuine inherence in a form which we may term logical inherence, according to which the emotional tonality is a part or aspect of the color or sound

---

faction, and suffering, were wholly restricted to any class of nerves; for this sense is scarcely distinguishable from life itself as expressed in awareness. The optic-nerve centers are all that color feelings require.

[18] DeWitt H. Parker, *The Analysis of Art* (New Haven: Yale University Press, 1926), pp. 75-76. Reprinted by kind permission of the publishers.

quality, and may be distinguished from it by abstraction but not otherwise separated from it. According to this conception, redness without emotional tone can neither be conceived nor exist, just as a red devoid of spatial character or of a certain intensity is a nonsensical concept. The significance of the doctrine of inherence is hardly more than that it paves the way for a perception of the logical identity of the two factors held to be necessarily connected. For since, as we have seen in previous chapters, the sense quality is a logically saturated entity and, since nothing over and above its mere quality (as saturated yellow, e.g.), its extensity, and intensity can be given as in it, the inherence theory is perhaps the most untenable of all. Moreover, it fails to meet the aesthetic requirements which motivate the very admission of aesthetic feelings as actual facts. These feelings are facts because aesthetic experience reports them as observed. But as observed they are not merely inherent, i.e., further characters additional to the redness of the red patch. The two do not merely observably inhere in the same surface, but they are given as one, as not really distinct at all. The sense of distinctness arises when we drop the aesthetic attitude and adopt that of practical manipulation and sign-reading ("this is red" meaning it has the character possessed by danger signals, or blood, or the book I have been seeking, etc.). That this is true, writers on aesthetics frequently admit, but they insist that the reports of aesthetic experience must be explained or analyzed and not simply accepted. For aesthetic observation quality and feeling ("form" and "content") are not distinguishable —granted, says many a writer; but "theoretically," i.e., outside aesthetic observation, we may distinguish them. This contention amounts to this: the aesthetic observation of sense data, that is to say, by the best definitions of "aesthetic," maximally vivid and sustained direct intuition of sense data, discloses them much less as they, as intuitive data, really are than do certain hypothetical distinctions based upon the casual observations of non-aesthetic life![19] But, you object, the aesthetic attitude is not analytic, and knowledge requires analysis. Granted,

---

[19] Cf. Schopenhauer, *The World as Will and Idea*, Book III, § 36.

on both counts, but it remains true that the final test of analysis is observed fact, and that observation of sense data, as such, is aesthetic in proportion to its concentration. The question always is: Does the analysis fit the observed phenomena, when they are carefully, vividly, i.e., aesthetically, perceived? The answer which many aesthetic writers give to this question in regard to their own theory is, in effect, "No, intuition negates the facts asserted by our analysis." It seems to follow that we should try a different analysis and continue to do so until we find one which is perceptually verified. Any other attitude is dogmatic, not scientific. Mere inherence, in sum, is not the adequate solution of the sensation-feeling relationship.

The rôle of similarity in aesthetic expression has been recognized since Plato and Aristotle. Indeed, it was by the back doorway provided by this concept into the orthodox Greek doctrine of art as imitation that expressionism first appeared in aesthetics. Both Plato and Aristotle remarked upon the fact (as it seemed to them, and has seemed to many since) that, at least in one instance, that of music, there was a relation of imitation—that is to say, of similarity—between presented sense patterns and something apparently of a rather different order, the internal emotions of man. Musical sounds as copies or simulacra of feelings—this was the form in which expressionism emerged in Greek thought. The emergence was hardly complete; it was not clear what application could be made of the doctrine to arts other than those of music and the drama, and, moreover, there was, in the Platonic account of music as a language of the emotions, an ambiguity with respect to the crucial question of whether the resemblance to feelings could actually be predicated of the individual tones of the music or only of the patterns of rhythm or melody—that is to say, whether quality as well as structure was expressive.

The limitation of expression to structure may be called "formalism." The classic exponent is Hanslick. The formalistic theory is a perfect example of the artificial dichotomies, the oversimplifications, in which modern rationalism, decreasingly since the eighteenth century it is true, has delighted. The decisive objections are that in fact even the most perfectly single tones, colors, odors, do observably and vividly express; and that most of the arguments leading to the expressionist position are quite as relevant to qualities as to structures. Indeed, as we have already argued, coherence of aesthetic structure is, in certain cases at least, inexplicable except in terms of the expressiveness of the elements entering into it. And, further, the inclusion of any feelings at all in the aesthetic whole of attention implies integration, and hence similarity of those feelings with all other elements. Thus the formalistic restriction of emotional affinities to structural aspects is the attempt to canalize the necessarily all-pervasive blending of aesthetic factors.

The stress upon similarity is distinguishable only in degree from the identity theory. For by this latter we mean that a certain subclass of feeling tones is the class "sensory qualities," but that the classification of the latter in this manner signifies merely that the similarities between them and the classes of feeling tones not identical with them are more important than the differences. It is impossible that the species of a genus should possess no characters peculiar to it by which it is distinguished from all other species of the genus. Moreover, in saying that the aesthetic feelings are identically sensations, we do not mean that there are no feelings involved in such an experience which are distinct from sensations. We mean that there is a certain objectified portion of the affective content which as objectified is sufficiently distinct from the subjective and bodily feelings to appear at a casual glance to compel classification as a distinct genus, but which a closer inspection reveals as connected with the internal feelings by such thoroughgoing affinities that it is more descriptive of the facts to employ the single genus "feeling." This is the more apparent in that the very character of objectivity by which, above all, the sensory feelings are distinguished may be described in terms of distinctions (namely, of social reference) illustrated even by the most subjective feelings. Finally, the tendency pervading most aesthetic descriptions to ascribe the affectivity of sensations to a factor distinct from them, but yet in some more or less paradoxical or illusory confusion or identity with them, can be explained as the manner in which the real generic affinities of sensations and unexternalized feelings force themselves upon the attention of close observers but, owing to the failure to distinguish sharply the various factors involved, and the strong materialistic tradition, fail to achieve consistent analysis. Some of the feeling is connected with the sensations by association; but, further, some of the feeling simply is the sensations; while the doctrine of externalized feeling projected, superimposed, upon sensation is the unanalyzed blend of at least these two truths.

The decisive facts, in sum, are these: (1) Certain of the aesthetic feelings are given as pervading the object, in a sense logically absurd unless they are given as identical with the secondary qualities which likewise are observed to pervade the object. (2) Further, aesthetic coherence demands (*a*) that all feelings which are not identical with sense qualities should be interblended with and similar to them, and (*b*) that sense qualities should possess similarities to one another which they seem in fact to lack unless interpreted as feeling tones. (3) Finally, the attentional supremacy of the sensory complex characteristic of aesthetic contemplation requires that the vivid enjoyment experienced should be in part identical with that sensory content, since nothing can attract and hold the attention in the presence of strong feeling except strong feeling. Emotional disturbances not actually inherent in the sensations and stronger than those which are form some of the most frequent preventives of genuine aesthetic perception. (Is it not because of them that artists frequently deny the emotional character of pure aesthetic experience?)

The synthesis of the foregoing considerations is found only in the doctrine that the entire warp and woof of aesthetic intuition, its sole content, is feeling, a part of which is identically the sensory qualities.

This is exactly the meaning, or at least part of the meaning, of the formula: art = intuition = expression. However, many interpreters of Croce's doctrine, including Croce himself, deduce various more or less paradoxical consequences from the formula, which contains, in fact, a possible ambiguity. To say the immediately intuited is "identically" the emotionally felt, the expressive, is to assert either: (a) I intuit only my own emotional states; or (b) I intuit only emotional states (Croce's "sheer emotion absolutely identified with the most lucid imagery") but these are not merely my own emotions but those of a not-myself, become also mine by immediate sympathy. (This not-self I take to be in all cases chiefly the bodily cells as having their own feelings.) Now it is against (a), which seems to be Croce's own position, that such critics of Croce as Carritt mainly direct their shafts. But the difficulty, urged by Carritt, that there could be no communication of feeling, since there would (by [a]) be nothing objective in which the feeling could be embodied, no contact with a real physical world common to all, falls away entirely if expressionism is interpreted in a roughly Leibnizian rather than in a Berkeleian fashion, i.e., if position (b) is accepted. (For the bodily cells, in their turn, prehend the wider physical environment.) Carritt's own conclusion[20]—sense objects embody feeling because God so constructed them—is to me a pure evasion, not because it is theological, but because the first problem to be solved is what is the phenomenal relation between sense and feeling, not what power established this relation.

It is curious that the most plausible explanation of Croce's preference of (a) in contrast to (b) is his bias against all transcendence, especially theological. Now (b) is the complete denial of materialism, or the assertion that the structure as well as the quality of existence is spiritual; while (a) is the concession to materialism that physical reality cannot be loved for its own sake. It matters little whether this denial means the denial that matter is spiritual or the denial that it, as distinct from our, or God's, perception of it, exists at all (except that the latter denial is more manifestly false); in either case the essential "vision" which Croce rightly says is aesthetic experience is negated; for this vision is of a mode of reality at once physical and spiritual and the two absolutely in one. Surely it is Leibniz (or White-

---

[20] E. F. Carritt, *The Theory of Beauty* (New York, 1914). A similar view is suggested by L. A. Reid, *A Study in Aesthetics* (London, 1930).

head), and not the Berkeley-Hegel group of idealists, who comes closest to explaining what such a reality must be. On the other hand, Croce's defense of the "identity" of feeling and the intuition of sense content, being based on extensive experience, as well as on vast knowledge of the aesthetic literature, deserves consideration on its merits and entirely apart from any prejudice for or against the Berkeleian subjectivism in which he seems to have entangled it, but which it by no means necessarily implies.[21]

### SECTION 25. QUALITY AND PATTERN

If, as is the doctrine of this book, a color or sound has, in addition to its associated affectivities, an intrinsic affective character, there is one class of men at least who might have been expected to discover this. I refer to artists, who more than other men are directly concerned with the mutual relations of feelings and sensations. Yet discussion with such persons elicits the fact that although the "emotional effects" of colors or of sounds is of interest to them, this interest, in the sense in which it would be most directly relevant to our problem, is a subordinate one. In the first place, in both painting and music, as well as in architecture, sculpture, dancing, etc.—in short, in all the arts—it is such formal elements as pattern or melody rather than single (visual or auditory) qualities that are of primary importance. Melody, tone color, rhythm, harmony, can be reproduced as substantially identical on a variety of instruments, or in a vari-

---

[21] Writers who adhere to a monistic standpoint in aesthetics include (besides Croce): Victor Basch, "Le maitre problème de l'esthétique," *Revue philosophique*, XCII, 1-26; also *Essai critique sur l'esthétique de Kant* (1896), pp. 73-103; Etienne Souriau, *L'avenir de l'esthétique* (Paris, 1929); Lascelles Abercrombie, *Toward a Theory of Art* (London, 1922); Louis Grudin, *Primer of Aesthetics* (New York, 1930); Paul Moos, *Moderne Musikästhetik in Deutschland* (1902), and *Die deutsche Ästhetik der Gegenwart* (1919); B. Bosanquet, *Three Lectures on Aesthetics* and *History of Aesthetics*.

The authors of the famous theory of *Einfühlung*, Th. Lipps (*Aesthetik*) and Volkelt (*System der Aesthetik* [2d ed.]; Munich, 1927), are dualists whose concessions to monism are so far reaching that, as Moos shows (in the second of the above-mentioned works), the only hope of ridding their assertions of inconsistency is to eliminate the dualistic aspect. It then appears that the only important mistake committed by this school was to assign to additional functions an achievement (the objectification of feeling) already competently performed by the mere act of sensing itself, indeed constituting its essential nature.

ety of keys; that is, the forms in question depend upon the relative or comparative character of the elements, not upon any absolute qualities of each. Moreover, the "effect" of the single elements themselves depends upon such relational properties as contrast, opposition, or harmony. In one picture red may seem rude, violent, restless, annoying; in another the same red may appear rich, dignified, and pleasing—all seems to depend upon the balance and relief afforded by the other colors. For the painter, the emotionality of colors is a matter of the dynamics of interaction set up when masses of color are simultaneously perceived. In music we find that attempts to state the emotional qualities of the several instruments of an orchestra, or of the several keys, or of a particular pitch, all prove oversimplifications in the face of the alterations produced by melody, rhythm, and harmony. An unpleasant, harsh discord in one melodic context may be delicious in another, etc. As for architecture, sculpture, dancing, here time and rhythm seem almost all-important and all-powerful in determining aesthetic meaning.

To the extent of this subordination of the single element to the total pattern, the artist is prejudiced against any attempt to discover an intrinsic aesthetic character in the elements taken singly.

And yet the artist is not really against us.[22] For the dependence of a given color for its aesthetic "effect" upon the color context, so far as this dependence is a fact, is thoroughly compatible with the view that the color in its qualitative identity is an aesthetic feeling. Here an ambiguity must be removed. In saying that the "same" color in different situations acquires diverse meanings, we must be careful not to mean merely the same physical pigment. For the assumption that variation in contrast leaves the relation of seen color to physical stimulus totally unaffected is unsafe; the change may result in an alteration of the shade actually perceived. For instance, black against

[22] Ozenfant (*op. cit.*) regards the emotional aspect of colors and sounds as fixed associations, universal to the race, forming the "constants" of art. But it is clear that the constancy is his main conviction rather than any particular explanation—such as association—of this constancy.

white is a more intense or pure black than could possibly be perceived against a background of blue or brown. Those, therefore, who say that the aesthetic quality of a color taken in pure isolation is indeterminate do not thereby establish a duality of color quality and aesthetic quality, for the color quality in pure isolation is also indeterminate if not inconceivable.

Abstracting from this difficulty, let us suppose that yellow is a gay or happy color; this implies that, other things being equal, we should be exhilarated by it. Suppose, however, that in a prevailingly somber picture a large mass of strong yellow is introduced, without due regard to balance, transition, mediation, and the like. The yellow may then affront us as out of place; it may be felt as violent rather than as cheering or joyous. Here it is above all to be noted that no amount of misplacing of yellow can so far alter its character as to transform its good cheer into the feeling of sheer negativity, of deathlike evil, which is characteristic of black. In spite of loose statements to the contrary, no such complete variability is demonstrable. Yellow may appear hateful, but its hatefulness, so far as it is objective feeling at all, is emotionally far different, in any circumstances, from that of black, under any circumstances. For the proof of this statement I can only send the reader to experience, to the study of works of art. He must use his own eyes, and not be content to repeat what he has somewhere read or carelessly conjectured. And now I ask how better explain the objectionableness of yellow out of place than to say that its light-heartedness may often jar too sharply with the prevailing melancholy of the picture; similarly, how better explain the satisfying character of yellow in the proper context than by saying (or perceiving) that its gaiety is balanced, and completed, yet not too brutally opposed, by the more serious characters of the remaining colors, so that in the whole something like the total of life's emotional possibilities is shown, just as in a Shakespearean tragedy. Black needs white as the villain needs the hero. This principle renders aesthetic relativity intelligible. And finally, in regard to the objection that yellow has a varying emotional character according to the individual or to the mood of the moment, has anyone, we may ask, failed to encounter the experience of reacting negatively to a positive emotion of which, as such, he is conscious? Has the gaiety of children never intensified the moroseness of adults or of the less happy among the children themselves? Has the merriment of others never appeared as cruel, impudent, immoderate, hateful? In short, how can a demonstrated variation in our emotional (subjective) "reaction" to something which we experience disprove the assumption that that to which we thus variously react is itself perceived as a nonvarying (objectified) emotion? Need we—indeed, can we intelligibly—assume the absolute simplicity of emotional structure which this mode of argument requires?

The further factors that serve to explain aesthetic relativity or variations of taste, together with the undeniable importance of the supersensory factors of learning and discrimination, without the assumption of a dualism of sense and feeling, may be summarized as follows:

In the first place, some of these variations may be explained by undetected defects in the sense organs—such as color-blindness or partial tone-deafness.[23] In the second place, even with normality of organs, there are vast differences in the quantity and distribution of attention upon which depend both the absolute and the relative vividness of sense data as well as the order in which they are brought into focus (as when one's gaze wanders about a picture, or one gives special heed at a symphony concert now to the violins, now to the wind instruments, now to the drums). One may attend to some part and scarcely sense others at all, or one may emphasize some part unduly, or one may miss much of the "meaning." But these errors produce alterations in the sheer sensory complex as given, alterations with respect to temporal sequence and order of vividness at least, if not slight alterations in the actual colors or tones intuited. Therefore these cases cannot be taken as proof that sense datum and meaning are distinct. Furthermore, all sensory

---

[23] In the present state of auditory theory, and in view of the mystery of octave quality, we are bound to be in some uncertainty concerning the equivalence of any two sets of ears.

emotions, to occur at all, must be integrated into the total emotional complex, inclusive of the more internal reactions, and of the intellectual feelings or ideas. Attention is itself thus an aesthetic adjustment. Complicated music which is not "understood" is also in the literal sense not, or not clearly, heard. Only if the whole being pulsates in emotional unison with an intricate pattern of sound feelings can attention consistently focus upon that pattern. The assumption that persons whose sense of the meaning of a piece of music differs can yet have the very same sense perception of the sounds is, so far as I know, devoid of all evidence. What is it but the uncritical acceptance of a notion accurate enough for the cruder purposes of everyday life as accurate enough also for science and for art? The painter and the philistine both perceive a table as a table—therefore they have the same sense perception of it! But the least investigation will show how vastly more complete and sustained is the sense experience of the artist.

In the second place, although the value of an aesthetic experience is in part quite literally localized in the sensations, it is of course not exclusively realized in them. Granting that sensing is in itself a certain quantity of feeling, it still does not follow that it is a quantity sufficient for full aesthetic satisfaction. The usual view that the sensing is a stimulus to feeling, which is partly determined also by the past experience of the individual, is true even on the affective theory of sensation. For it is clear that feelings can be associated with and give rise to feelings. One sorrow tends to recall another; a joyous mood can give rise to a succession of happy thoughts. The fulness of the aesthetic experience is due to the enriching of sense-feelings with a background of reactive feelings such that the former are felt as representative of the latter in the manner of samples. Thus the joy of the bobolink's intoxicated carol is felt as illustrative of the joy of life and love in the summer sunshine—it reverberates in the memory and imagination, awakening echoes from all that is akin to it. This enhancement through kindred experiences is the real "appreciation," which may require the preparation of culture, or the appropriate strain of temperament. It is no use for the musician to weave delicate shades of feeling into his pattern of notes if the listener's emotional habits are such as to emphasize less fine or quite incongruous emotional contrasts. The listener in that case will in fact not listen, even if he should try. Alien thoughts will bear the current of full attention irresistibly elsewhere.[24] And in so far as he does listen, he will not provide that amplification of relevant imagining and response whereby the finite morsel of sense feeling becomes fused with the infinite or inexhaustible constituency of related feelings for which it stands. Thus the sense quality is of value neither wholly for itself nor wholly for its associations, but as with flowers from the beloved, the intrinsic beauty is enhanced immeasurably by the symbolic import. If the sensations were to be valued not at all for themselves, they would not even be sensed. Just as truly as they are seen, they are grasped as naked, direct values (good or evil); but if they were valued wholly for themselves, we should have become creatures limited to our external sensory functions, a state unrealized even in the lower animals. Nothing can be valued wholly for itself, not even the dearest of friends, nor yet wholly as a means, not even a brass tack. The person is useful as well as good, the instrument is aesthetically expressive as well as convenient. Always there is a direct grasp of life fusing into other life, of end-in-itself in one with our end, and in one with the organic and infinite whole of ends, the vaguely intuited cosmic society. Valuation is social and mystical; there is only a variation in the degree of explicitness which it attains in respect to these characteristics.

Still another cause of inconstancy in aesthetic evaluation is the rôle of associated sensory images. There is, in fact, a subtle blending of perceptual and imaginative colors and forms in the seeing of a picture or a statue. Just as, in reading, a missing letter or even an entire word will be supplied by "apperceptive" activity, so in all sense experience, the sensory material intuited is only partially determined by the external stimulus. The fusion of images from other senses, touch and kinesthetic with visual, for example, is also a well-known and ever present factor. The very consciousness of the third dimension which distinguishes painting from flat design is in part injected into the pic-

---

[24] See the essay by Charles Myers in Max Schoen's *Effects of Music*.

ture by such associations, and it is known that savages often quite fail to mobilize the imagery required, and so find a painting unintelligible. In music the retention of auditory sensations in memory, and their anticipation on the basis of past experience, are of course vital to appreciation. Thus probably much of the emotional variability which is regarded as due to an inconstancy of association between affective and merely sensory factors—the latter assumed as constant—really involves variations in the sensory material itself, that is to say, in the emotional material in its objectified phases.

The true rôle of learning, i.e., individually acquired associations, may be illustrated in two opposite aspects from the sphere of music. On the one hand, we are often told that the most arresting and stirring music is that which we have heard from early childhood (the similar and even more startling effect of odors freighted with associated experiences is well known). From this one may argue for the acquired or associational status of aesthetic meaning. But one can also argue in an opposite direction, toward the conclusion that in childhood and youth one is less distracted by practical and intellectual obsessions—in short, by "associations"—from attention to the immediate savor of experiences, and derives therefore a more vivid impression of their aesthetic character. The associations which carry us back to an early hearing of the music carry us back also to an experience when we listened in complete absorption to the sounds, precisely because of lack of associations and powerful thought habits such as now tempt us to stray from our sensations into sophisticated more or less irrelevant channels—in short, a time when by the grace of the Creator of sense organs we really heard the music. But, on the other hand, when confronted with the most complicated forms of music, a child, a savage, a musically uncultivated person, or even one trained in the music of another culture will be unable at first to enjoy the sounds.[25] The

[25] Youtz says: "The factors in style are all .... matters which may be seen and heard. If beheld for the first time they may require a good deal of observation before they are grasped, but they need not be referred to the past for interpretation. The work of art is actually self-explanatory, though we may have to spend many hours before the explanation becomes apparent unless we start with a clue to its dominant forms. In relatively simple art, such as ceramics, for example, we can grasp with delight something

reason is that no such person is equipped with the habits of rapid auditory adjustment, of lightning-swift survey of form (aided by previous experience of similar forms), consequent anticipatory preparation for the next phrase, memory of the preceding, and just distribution of emphasis (localized attention) without which no man can steadily and clearly audit the notes as a pattern of sensations in their entirety. Furthermore, on the monistic hypothesis, it is impossible to attend to the notes except in so far as the mind stands ready to synthesize or fuse them into a total emotional integration, involving the entire conscious being, with which they are congruent. No one can listen to complex music without thinking. But there are patterns of thought which are so far homogeneous with the patterns of sound that thinking them is little more than, or fuses largely with, the acts of attentional adjustment, memory, and anticipation, by which alone the sounds can be heard.[26] So likewise there are associated feelings whose function is to form a frame into which the audited feelings (the sounds as heard) can merge without loss of vividness. The art of aesthetic appreciation is to "associate" with the object solely the images and reactions whose affective content will permit the sensory content to remain in the focal center rather than such as will displace it therefrom; and—this is the same thing in other words—which will find the supreme illustration of their own "spirit" in that sensory content—as all the spirit of a piece of music is concentrated in its principal theme, or the subordinate parts of a picture in its central areas—rather than such as will be merely joined to the sense datum by an associative link. Marriage through affinity with, and under condition of subordination to, the sense perceptions—this is the sole legitimate destiny of all that is more than sense perception, more than just the achievement of maximum attention to the stimulus, in the experience of art. To this statement I believe many artists would subscribe.

---

largely exotic. But in complex forms, such as painting or architecture or music, a first impression will hardly resolve them unless we already know the stylistic language." (*Sounding Stones of Architecture* [New York: W. W. Norton & Company, Inc., 1928], p. 245). Reprinted by permission of the publishers.

[26] Cf. Schoen, *op. cit.*, p. 58.

# CHAPTER VI

# THE DIMENSIONS OF EXPERIENCE

\*\*

*It is not so much from counting as from measuring, not so much from the conception of number as from that of continuous quantity, that the advantage of mathematical treatment comes. Number, after all, only serves to pin us down to a precision in our thoughts, which, however beneficial, can seldom lead to lofty conceptions, and frequently descends to pettiness. . . . . The excessive use of it must tend to narrow the powers of the mind. But the conception of continuous quantity has a great office to fulfill, independently of any attempt at precision. . . . . It is the direct instrument of the finest generalizations. . . . . By means of it, the greatest differences are broken down and resolved into differences of degree, and the incessant application of it is of the greatest value in broadening our conceptions.*

CHARLES S. PEIRCE

\*\*

### SECTION 26. DIMENSIONAL ANALYSIS IN SCIENCE

IF WE consult the most indubitably successful of the positive sciences, we find that a conspicuous cause of their success lies in the constant use which they make of the idea of dimensional variation—of differences which in principle are graduated or continuous. It matters not at all whether discontinuities—"quanta"—are involved. The principle of continuous variation is equally vital, since the very idea and magnitude of the quanta can be stated only in terms of it. Mere discreteness is not to be imagined in the physics of space-time. In short, it is the historical fact that man has begun to understand something when he has found a way to geometrize it. This is the immortal insight of Plato, rediscovered by Leibniz and Peirce.

Philosophers have generally supposed that all distinctions among things which lend themselves to geometrical or dimensional treatment belong to the special sciences, leaving for philosophy itself only irreducibly "qualitative," i.e., absolute, differences. This implies that philosophy is irreducibly unscientific, for absolute differences offer nothing to the understanding, and there is furthermore no criterion for their verification in experience. (Let the reader ask himself what an absolute difference would be like, if he were to meet one in experience, and by what mark he would recognize its presence.) It also implies that the world is not the coherent whole which philosophy itself has been inclined to posit. On all counts it seems better to accept the principle of Parmenides, Leibniz, Kant, Cournot, Peirce, Montague—to mention some exceptions to the philosophic neglect of continuity—as the guiding idea in philosophical as it is in scientific inquiry.

We are often told that the question "What is it?" has been superseded by the more scientific "How does it behave?" But it is overlooked that the former question is elliptical for the colloquial "What is it like?" and that this again needs expansion into "With what groups of other things and in what logical manner does it form dimensional systems of graduated differences?" These dimensions include others besides those specifiable exclusively in terms of behavior; and the inquiry concerning these hyperphysical likenesses and differences among things is a legitimate appeal to observation and logical analysis. It can never rightfully be cut off by a priori dogmas.

That the physical variables by virtue of their uniquely public character are scientifically crucial need not be denied. Indeed, it is to be emphasized that only when all qualitative dimensions have been translated into behavioristic correlates will we have effective intellectual control of them. The affective continuum is potentially a physical fact if it is a fact at all. With "methodological materialism" in this sense its supporters need have no quarrel.

SECTION 27. THE SOCIAL CONTINUUM

If the principle of continuity holds, then the difference between myself and my neighbor is a difference of degree; and there will be some contents in my experience which are more and others which are less "mine" rather than "thine." The latter class of contents must include at least the more external of the sensory qualities, especially those of color and sound. But philosophers and psychologists have done their best to derive the doctrine of sensation from the least social of our sensory experiences, and on the basis of the non-social theory of sensation so derived they have then deduced that since the objective, i.e., sensory, contents are private, wholly unshared, therefore the less objective contents are still more certainly not directly shared, and so nothing is directly shared and all is wholly private—in the face of the fact that for physics a man's body is most certainly far from possessing such absolute privacy. After this valuable result has been reached, it is then necessary to explain how social communication, with its identity of meanings and interests, does take place, and, to date, the problem remains one of the great dividers of philosophical opinion. If we begin first by recognizing that the self-identity and distinctness of individuals is not a matter of absolutes, proceed by inferring that my neighbor is therefore only partially other than or external to myself, finally approach experience on the definite lookout for social community as permeating experience, we may find that the non-social doctrine of sense data is false, that therefore the problem of how minds communicate is in principle and quite obviously soluble empirically.

But other and more obvious grounds of the priority of the social principle can be given. For example, the social continuum is one in which the nature of the two opposite poles is particularly clear. The psycho-physical continuum, for example, is indefinitely more elusive, so much so that it is far from obvious how there can be any kinship between mind and an electron. It is, on the contrary, quite obvious that there is a kinship of quality between one person and another, and that this fact is more deeply rooted in its certainty than the inference to the nature of a physical substance. Sociality is a clearer idea than psycho-physicality. Nor is it less rich in implications; for a social relation implies an environment, and in fact the social functions of man embrace in one way or another all his functions.

Doubtless the neglect of sociality is partly explicable on the ground of its logical complexity, from which has been inferred its derivative character. Combine two persons and you have sociality; therefore we should first simplify our problem by considering one person and his private non-social experience. This argument takes for granted a metaphysical premiss than which none could be more fundamental. Is sociality a derivative result of the combining of privacies? Is a conscious individual related to other conscious individuals only by what from the logical point of view is an accident? Is experience ever at any point non-social—for example, is physical perception of a stone a non-social experience? You may say, "obviously, yes." But this "obviously" rests upon the assumption that you have a wholly clear idea of social, and a wholly clear perception of your perception of the stone; for the judgment of the absolute disparity of two ideas (aside from its logical absurdity) presupposes all this. Now, that you have such a clear idea and such a clear perception of your perception is very far from obvious.

From the standpoint of continuity, what one must say is that the perception of the stone may be one in kind but very different in degree as compared with experiences generally recognized as social. The sociality of the stone experience need not be zero in order to escape ordinary observation. We must remember Faraday's principle, or the principle of the most favorable conditions for observation.[1] The habit of assuming that philosophical questions are essentially questions of all or nothing, rather than of degree, has resulted in the wholesale violation of this rule, so vital to success in the sciences.

Instead of defining the social as a complex of too high a degree to represent the primordial principle of mind, we ought rather to define it in such a way as to allow for variations in complexity along as wide a range of degrees as possible. Let us mean by social feeling merely "feeling of feeling." Let anyone then show that this concept involves a complexity of structure higher than that inherent in being as such, which, unless Parmenides

[1] "The discovery [of diamagnetism] was probably due to Faraday's habit of not regarding as final any negative result of an experiment until he had brought to bear upon it the most powerful resources at his command" (S. P. Thompson, *Michael Faraday* [New York, 1898], p. 184).

is a flawless metaphysician, is surely a degree above zero. If it appears a paradox to say that feeling of feeling is as fundamental as mere feeling, then it should be a paradox to say that being, related to being, is as fundamental as mere being. Yet who doubts that this is the case? The attempt to treat the social aspect of mind in its widest sense as in any fashion derivative from the purely private, or the latter as in any wise independent of the former, belongs with all attempts to treat relations as secondary features of the universe. It is time that such attempts be dropped. It is time that we shook ourselves free forever from all doctrines that treat the private as anything but an aspect of the relation of mind to mind. It is not enough to yield inch by inch to facts exhibiting the social character of mental growth or of the basic human desires. The point is that there are two possible views: either mind or awareness as such is logically dependent upon other mind or awareness, or it is not. The latter view has been tried. It has led to all the paradoxes of epistemology, and to a disastrous attempt to found duty upon self-interest. The other view has scarcely been tried at all.

### SECTION 28. THE ULTIMATE DIMENSIONS

The framework of all qualitative analysis is accordingly to be sought in the dimensions of the social situation as such. "Dimensions" is meant in the mathematical sense of independent variables. In the present application it denotes the respects in which the social situation admits distinctions of greater and less, or is a matter of degree. Thus if we analyze sociality into its main distinguishable factors or aspects, we have then only to discover the possibility of variations in the degree of emphasis upon each factor, to have demonstrated the existence of dimensions of sociality.

The most obvious distinction involved in all social feeling is that between self and other. So far as it is the self which is felt, the feeling may be termed, in a certain non-moral or technical sense, selfish; so far as the feeling concerns an other, it may be termed other-regarding. Now are not all possible applications of this distinction relative, matters of degree? The feeling of

## § 28 THE DIMENSIONS OF EXPERIENCE 195

self is not an absolute thing, which is either simply there or not there, but on the contrary a factor fluctuating endlessly between vaguely demarcated extremes of vividness or centrality and dimness or unfocused indirectness of attention. So with the consciousness of an other. The whole aspiration of life amounts to the desire of increasing the intensity of both of these poles, without detriment to either. Here, then, are at once two dimensions of social feeling, according as feeling is predominantly self- or other-regarding, and according as the contrast between these two poles of consciousness is more or less explicit. There are all degrees of balance toward one side or the other and all degrees of quantity in the masses balanced.

Sociality, we have seen, implies a relation of at least two individuals, and individuality in the social sense means a certain freedom, or independence of action. Suppress the idea of activity, and the idea of the social situation becomes void of empirical content. Suppress striving, and you suppress the significance of pleasure and pain, of joy and sorrow, of grief, hope, and aspiration, of co-operation and the sharing in effort, surprise, disappointment, and fulfilment. What does not undergo and react cannot belong to the great community of socially continuous individuals. Here, then, is the dimension generated by the contrast of action and passion, the exertion and the sufferance of power or influence. Social activity involves always some degree of passivity toward the influence exerted by others, and equally does such passivity, however extreme, involve always a certain amount of activity.

In activity there is further a distinction of polarity—a distinction of the dynamically negative and positive. Pleasure and pain, joy and sorrow, love and hate, are expressions of this opposition. They may be reached from the concept of activity by the mediation of the idea of will as immediately conscious or felt striving.

In all of the foregoing, use is made of the concept of the degree or intensity with which a factor is present. This contrast of faint-intense presents at least the semblance of an additional dimension, for it appears that experience as a whole can vary along it, in some independence of the relative intensities of self as contrasted with other; activity, with passivity; positive, with negative.

Given the four grand dimensions of self-other, active-passive, positive-negative, faint-intense, the world of common experience and science, in its broadest outline, can be seen, I affirm, as a natural consequence.[2] It seems also clear that all of these variables have inalienable behavioristic implications, and that consequently they are not purely private, subjective, or ineffable. If such things as sense qualities can be described in terms of them, then it is not true that the redness of one person's experience might be different from that of another's without any possibility of verifying the fact.

### SECTION 29. SPACE: THE PRIMARY QUALITIES

Space and time are aspects of the contrast between the self and another. We shall consider here only space.

The self is here, the other is there—his realized otherness is his thereness. How else (apart from temporal differences) could that otherness be a realized fact? As for nearness and farness, the near is that which is socially apprehended in a more intimate fashion, or with greater vividness than the far. One may show this by various experiments.

In the first place, the mere fact that nearness means greater fulness of detail proves that the near is the more intimate and

---

[2] The three qualitative dimensions above considered are somewhat similar to those proposed by Burlton Allen (*Pleasure and Instinct* [New York: Harcourt, Brace & Co., 1930], p. 299) in the following words (reprinted by permission of the publishers):

"There are, I would suggest, three forms which the mental life can take..... Each of these makes up a 'dimension' in which a number of degrees can exist between two opposites. These are as follows:

"1. The dimension moving between success and failure, effectiveness and non-effectiveness, the smooth and obstructed working out of the instinctive conations.

"2. That moving within degrees of activity and passivity, in respect to which we feel ourselves more or less self-directed.

"3. That of the differing depth or intensity with which the conscious self is engaged in the reaction, the result being that the total experience appears on the one hand as in varying degrees, vivid, important, exciting, on the other as deadened, trivial, dull."

The view of the dimensions of feeling set forth by Harlow and Stagner in their article in the *Psychological Review* (XXXIX [1932], 570-89) has also considerable analogy to the doctrine of this section.

vivid, as in the distance details grow faint and disappear. Again a dear friend when recollected as dear seems closer than he physically is, and an intense pain in the foot, which by its intensity becomes more united to the self, closer than a faint one. It tends to shift the emotional center of gravity toward itself, to become more a reactive, less an objective, feeling. In these and innumerable other ways one may verify the statement that space is simply the form of social externality (otherness) as such. The spatial depth of perception is its social objectification. The zero of perceived depth is one's self, the maximum or infinite of depth likewise the infinite of social independence. Depth is epistemological—it can only be understood if objectivity to the mind and distinction from it are relative only, admitting degrees. The direct consciousness of this degree of intimate union with the self is "near" and "far" as percepta. The dimensions of up and down, right and left, on the contrary, do not have self at one end and extreme social independence at the other; for in their case the self is midway, or neutral. The self is no more right than left, or up than down. These relations may hold between terms which are equally objectified relatively to us. Depth-distance gives us distinction, independence, active individuality, yet social *rapport*, with respect to others; but up and down, right and left, give those others the same independence and *rapport* among themselves, but all this for our perception. Without them the most complex social situation which could be adequately perceived would be dual, and this dual situation itself could not be adequately objectified. To see my relation to the other objectively is to see it as one in which, to the eye of the disinterested beholder, we are both on the same level. But depth is essentially egocentric and interested. The two poles are not balanced in their relation to the observer. Only the cross-dimensions can give such balance. All the dimensions accordingly express depth or social distinctness, but if depth for me is the "first" dimension, then the remaining or "cross"-dimensions are depth for or between others, their mutual depth as a fact for me or as terminus of my depth. Unobjectified and objectified depth, depth *simpliciter* and depth as its own terminus—in these two ideas lies the secret of space as directly experienced.

From the many questions which immediately suggest themselves in regard to the foregoing brief account of space—for instance, the question why the number of cross-dimensions should be neither more nor less than two—we here abstract. One question only may be touched upon, namely: What is the difference between apparent or perceived and real or physical spatial relations? The answer is that it is the difference between apparent and real social relations. The latter must be inferred from and conceived in the same general terms as the former. These terms are provided by the concept of "feeling of feeling." Space, together with time, is the structural articulation of this "of."[3]

It is notable that the individualities of geometrical figures can be unambiguously specified in social terms. Thus a triangle is the only mode of social grouping in which three individuals may share alike in the same relationship to the group as a whole (may have their depth relations terminate in the depth relations of the others in the same wise). A square fulfils the same conditions for four, and so on for all regular polygons. A circle has the unique property that an unlimited number of individuals may be so grouped that none has a favored position (other things being equal) to the whole group. Herein is the merit of a circular dining-table. A straight line is the opposite extreme: only two persons can have impartial group relations along such a line. If there are three persons, two of them will have the advantage or disadvantage of being on the outside of the group (being in the unobstructed depth of but one of the two others). Similar remarks apply to three-dimensional figures.

These considerations have relevance to the old mystery of the aesthetic individualities of spatial forms. It is an axiom of all artistic work that for a given "effect" only a certain given form will serve. Individual associations are not in practice assumed as relevant. Now if a geometrical form is nothing but a type of

[3] See A. N. Whitehead, *Process and Reality* (New York: Macmillan, 1930), Part IV, and, for a simpler account, *Science and the Modern World* (New York: Macmillan, 1925), pp. 90 ff.

social situation, this irreducible meaningfulness is intelligible. But—perhaps you will object—what has the perception of a simple design attended by no thought of social groupings and dinner parties to do with the significance of social-group types as such? I answer that perception has its own form of the social relation, that what we are attempting is the widest possible generalization of that relation, and that while it does not compel us to use "social" in a Pickwickian sense, it does compel us to use it in a subtle sense—one which has meaning only in view of rather careful observation of the facts.

Such a fact is this. A perceived color is a feeling felt objectively, as socially other than one's own feelings. In addition, it is always felt as in contrast or otherness to other colors (feelings) given or imagined simultaneously. Now in making a given color area one's special object of attention, in singling it out as something individual and distinct, one is on the way to feeling it as a full-fledged or high-grade organism of feeling, as a genuinely social other to one's self (cf. the protocols of von Allesch's or Huber's or Bullough's subjects). But in thus individualizing it, one has not, as a rule, wholly lost consciousness of its color-environment, the neighboring color-patches. If the first color or organic pattern of colors is in the center or focus of attention, the others are in the "fringe." This fringe, as Gestalt psychology insists, forms part and parcel of the color in the center. This is shown by the fact that to render the latter a completely distinct and independent object of attention is impossible, and the nearer we approach to it, the more we lose the original character of the color so attended to. Even if but one color seems to be apprehended, there is an apperceptive mass which supplies the contrast, and in this case also the contrast with one's self tends to be emphasized and to receive a social form. And certainly if a spatial form is perceived, it is defined by a plurality of colors, each of which has a degree of feeling individuality or organization above zero and a degree of overlapping or interfusion with the others above zero. This is equivalent to the single assertion that the degree of sociality of the situation is above zero. Moreover, the same laws of social grouping which constitute space hold here. The farther apart two colors are, or the more depth there is between them, the fainter is their emotional intermixture, and the more nearly they reach the ideal of absolute independence, metaphysical "outsideness" or sheer diversity of being, which common sense, with its usual callousness to questions of accuracy, assumes is already reached by their mere occupancy of different regions of space.

The upshot of the foregoing is that the puzzle of the relation between primary and secondary qualities is in principle solved. On the one hand, we seem to have sheer structure; on the other, sheer structureless simple qualities. Yet the age-old aesthetic fact is that in vivid experience this contrast is relativized, for here structure itself is felt as qualitative and qualities as life-expressive, and therefore implicative of the dimensions of contrast and complexity inseparable from life. The full solution is found, if at all, only in the recognition that feelings are socially structured intrinsically, and that in feeling the distinction between quality and relationship is a matter of emphasis only. "Love" is a quality and a structure of life in one; tear these aspects wholly apart and they and the entire universe become indeed ineffable and intelligence defeating. In the affective continuum, no distinctions not contrast effects are permissible, not even that between dimensions of the continuum and entities related by those dimensions.

As for mathematical space, in the sense of purely geometrical structures, these are the pure generalized types of possible social groupings as represented by groupings of symbols; and these latter are aesthetic, i.e., as shown above, sensory-social, patterns studied for their analogies with possible existential (causally efficacious) social groupings.

### SECTION 30. THE AFFECTIVE CONTINUUM

Our rule is to seek to reduce given distinctions to the mode of continuity. Now the contents of awareness are distinguished as a whole from the awareness which embraces them. We infer from the rule that we are to regard the difference between content and awareness as a matter of degree only, involving discoverable extremes and their intermediaries. What, then, is there in experience which appears to partake to some extent both of the character of awareness and of its contents, or which seems unmistakably of the stuff of consciousness and yet at the same time something in which consciousness terminates? The first evidence that a thing is intermediate in such fashion is that opinions differ more widely as to its inclusion or exclusion from a given class than is true of the other things classified; for clearly an intermediary can be assimilated as readily to one of its extremes as to the other, and where the idea of an intermediary is overlooked, such assimilation is likely to occur. The riddle in the present case is not hard to guess. There is a class of entities concerning which classifications as to subjective-objective do differ more uncertainly than with other classes. Indeed, these entities are treated both as contents and as modes of awareness itself. These are the aesthetic and affective characters of things. Santayana says that in aesthetic experience pleasure is objectified, appears as a content. Titchener agrees that affectivity extends at times over the whole of experience internal and external. Yet others deny all this, and only a very few thinkers admit that such characters are conceivable apart from awareness. There is a far less general agreement concerning the essential dependence of ordinary sensory qualities upon awareness. Now all these facts and many more are only what we should expect if affective qualities (those usually called such—for us all characters are affective) are in fact intermediate between pure subjective awareness and the most objective or purely "sensory" contents, such as red or green. How can we further test this hypothesis?

The proof of an intermediary is further intermediaries. Let us take the sweetness of the taste of sugar. Sweetness may not be admitted to be an affective quality, but it is idle to deny that it is easier to confuse it than the color red with such affective qualities as pleasantness and the like, for a whole section of language rests upon this confusion, if such it be. "Sweetness" is a value judgment about as often as not in ordinary parlance, if not more often than not. There is, then, some presumption that it is akin to affective qualities; but no less is it akin to the "neutral" sensations of color or sound, for while it appears absurd that a feeling of pleasantness should be disliked, it may sometimes happen, though with some appearance of paradox to most persons, that sweetness is disliked; while red may be liked or disliked without any very strong suggestion of paradox in either case. Suppose, then, for the moment that the sweetness of taste is intermediate in degree of subjectivity between a color and a feeling of pleasantness. Are there further intermediaries in either or in both directions? Take a pleasant organic sensation, as of the exquisite feeling of healthily tired muscles in repose. Surely this feeling is more obviously inconceivable as a fact outside of consciousness than is a color.

Consider a pain. A pain is not infrequently considered a sensation in the proper psycho-physical sense. But this does not alter the fact that the classification "pleasure-pain" has always appeared a natural one. A pain, then, is perhaps more akin to genuine affectivity than is a taste, but is more nearly of the "neutrality" of taste than is pleasure. Let us consider pleasure itself. Does it lead to any further progress toward the subjective? Surely there are degrees of resemblance to the sensory in pleasure. For there are highly localized pleasures (and it is sensation that is local),[4] and there are pleasures that merge into what is called "joy," and which are scarcely distinguishable from the character of an awareness as a whole. From a state of ecstasy into which great music may throw us, appearing to color the entire warp and woof of our consciousness at the time, so that the very lights in the concert hall seem to be echoing with their twinkling brightness the joy which is in us, and all our thoughts, perceptions, and images seem held together by a bond of aesthetic enjoyment in no clear way distinguishable from the bond of awareness as a whole, from this all-pervasive joy down to the "sweetness" of a single violin note there is a vast series of intermediaries, with scarcely a gap of any magnitude.

Thus there appears to be no good reason why the distinction

[4] What account conventional dualistic psychology can give of the sex sensation-pleasure is hard to imagine.

of content and awareness should not be treated as continuous, with affectivity as the mediating concept. Let us call qualities of contents "content forms," and qualities characterizing awareness as a whole "awareness forms"; and let us regard awareness forms as the upper section of an ascending series of more and more subjective or comprehensive affective states, and content forms as the lower section, the more and more sharply localized and psychically distanced (socially individuated) members, of this series.

Is there anything "between" qualities from different senses, a color and a sound for example? If there is such a thing, it may be either another color or sound or else a character from still a third sense, say a smell. Between or intermediate means in some respect, that is to say as determining some line of variation. But such a line is a universal. Now psychology already admits a number of universals spanning the *verboten* chasm between classes of *sensa*. Such are the "attributes" of sensation: spatiality, temporality, intensity. If it can be shown that these are really lines of variation, that is to say admit of degree, so that it can have a verifiable meaning to speak of one sensation as more or less spatial or temporal than another, then we should find here one clue to the intermediaries we seek. Are the different senses equal with respect to spatiality or temporality? This is so far untrue that it has been disputed whether or not spatiality, at least, really is a universal attribute of sensation; and as for duration, it is so far diminished in much of our visual experience that the neglect of the category of time in most philosophy may not unplausibly be regarded as encouraged by the predominance of visual imagery over that from other senses. A color may be essentially a process, but who shall say that this is as obvious as it is that a sound is a process?[5] Surely there is a diminution of emphasis upon temporality in vision as compared to hearing. To find intermediaries in this case is not so easy, but I suggest that smell may be one.

[5] All the distinctive features of color as contrasted to sound, smell, etc., are less apparent in the phenomena of "depth" color, "light" color, and "shine," than in "surface" colors.

With such attributes as modes of graduated likeness we are in a position to interpret the ultimate meaning of the divisions among *sensa*. The attribute of spatiality alone accounts for an amazing portion of the differences. Imagine something resembling a temperature sensation—the sense of warmth, let us say—except that it is imagined as localized out there in space as is a color. Is there anything unfair or question-begging in this conception, or anything absurd; anything in the nature of space or of warmth as a quale which requires that that quale should be in one place rather than in another? Now in fact I do find for myself and—what is more to the point—there is evidence that the human race in general has found, that such a conception is perfectly possible. When I conceive of the warmth as out there where a color ordinarily is, I find that my conception is unmistakably that of the sort of color that would be called "warm," namely, a reddish or orange glow. Cold, on the other hand, would be a paler color, of what hue I am less certain. The same imagined metamorphosis of a smell or a sound into a color is equally feasible.

What is the quality of sweetness if not a pleasantness sharply localized on the tongue instead of vaguely suffused over a larger area of consciousness? True, some people dislike "sweets," but these produce a blend of sweetness with other tastes and smells, and it is this blend which is disliked. Or, if it is really the taste, say, of pure sugar which is considered insipid, this means that a small patch of rather mild pleasant feeling is found insignificant from the standpoint of experience as a whole, whereas an intrinsically unpleasant bitterness by providing a shock and foil may stimulate and enhance other reactions whose value outweighs that of mere sweetness. There is a similar value in cold showers and other not intrinsically agreeable sensory experiences. Value is enhanced by victory, dominance over its opposite. The cold sensation derived from ice-cream is in itself somewhat painful, as anyone who tries some made without flavor will find, but this negative affectivity enhances the positive feelings of taste and smell provided by the fruit juices, sugar, etc., as well as by the touch sensation of smoothness imparted by the creamy consistency. The Gestalt character of most of the values even of the despised chemical senses is commonly neglected, leading to the idea that the aesthetic attributes of color or sound combinations are something peculiar to the senses of vision and audition, whereas in fact the problems of gustatory preference involve the same principles of harmony, contrast, and dissonance which explain beauty in the higher senses. Even the principle of expression is not wholly absent. The analysis of what the taste of turnips expresses may be beyond me, but I know it does not express the sort of feelings I readily entertain, and that to like it very much I should have to have a fundamentally different personality, or a different olfactory nerve.

In considering these suggestions we must remember that the feelings identified with the sensory qualities mentioned are spatially localized and more or less externalized affectivities, distinguished as such from the more subjective kinds by the fact that they are given with more detachment from the self. They are given as feelings *for* rather than *of* one's self—in other words, as semisocialized feelings, on the way from the "I" to the "you." That such social objectification of feeling does not destroy its character as feeling is the presupposition of there being any genuinely social experience at all.

Consider a strong smell of a character no one would think to call fragrant, which none the less fascinates through its piquancy. Surely this pleasantness is very different from—in a way nearly the opposite to—the pleasantness of a genuine fragrance. The difference is irreducible by any associations and on our theory constitutes the difference between the fragrance as a datum and the piquant smell as a datum. Thus the smell of a skunk—which in moderate intensity may be enjoyed—is a bitter-like smell, a bitterness differently spatialized from that of the taste of strychnine, but plainly akin to it. In what respect? In respect to the negativity which is one with the negativity of suffering as opposed to pleasure, hate as opposed to love, darkness as opposed to light, the fundamental negativity which can be nothing else than the negativity of evil as opposed to good. Vary the spatialization of this factor and you have: sorrow, grief, unpleasantness, pain, sour or bitter in taste or smell, sad sounds, blackness, etc. Take positivity and you have: joy, pleasure, sweet tastes, fragrance, sweet sounds, joyful colors.

But of course other qualitative dimensions than that of positive-negative are required. Active-passive, and faint or dull (as opposed by intense or sharp), are the two additional ones we have suggested. Their application in some detail will be attempted in the next chapter.

There is, however, one argument against the assimilation of contents and awareness which deserves to be considered. This is based upon the contention that the chief characteristic of a mental state, or a psychic process, is the reverberation of the past in the present, i.e., memory, and that this characteristic is lacking to sense data.[6] Now it is to be granted that the presence of anything like memory in sense data is not obvious. Yet there are, I suggest, grounds for supposing this presence. Here as everywhere we should reject the invitation to look upon the question as a matter of absolutes. A color looks static, purely contemporaneous, but does not a sound exhibit itself as rather plainly processional in character? And what can this mean if not that as given it includes a history—and what is this inclusion if not the inherence of a bit of memory in each present state of the sound? Indeed, does not the sense of musical relevance of a note to its predecessors enter into and alter the quality of the note? It is true that owing to their relative simplicity sense qualities cannot exhibit such an elaborate and explicit structure, temporal or otherwise, in their inner natures as can the more subjective aspects of experience. But this simplicity is due to vagueness, to our inability to analyze immediate intuitions except in crude terms. And the whole argument begs the question in that it supposes that a sense quality can be thought of as determinate without reference to its context, including the entire subjective side of experience with its explicit memories and other functions, whereas, as we have seen (sec. 4), only a generalization of the quality is independent of context. Finally, time as a continuum excludes non-processional qualities (see next section).

[6] See H. H. Price, *Perception* (London, 1932), pp. 120 ff.

## SECTION 31. VAGUENESS: THE EVOLUTION OF QUALITIES

In order to account for the emergence of new qualities in the world-process, which without such emergence would scarcely be a process, we must introduce a dimension of variation which was at best only hinted at in preceding sections. This is the dimension of degree of definiteness or specificity. When a color is seen by means of the peripheral part of the retina, it is not identifiable as any particular chroma, but neither is it that definitely non-chromatic quality called "gray." It is rather a chromatically indeterminate quality, and this indeterminateness is its quality. It is natural that thinkers in search of clarity and definiteness in their concepts should refuse to recognize the category of indefiniteness as expressing not only our own lamentable deficiency but the very dimension of cosmic creation. There has been no more persistent fallacy than this of supposing that the objects of inquiry must be clothed in an absolutely definite garb. It is true that the principle of excluded middle must be taken seriously; but the question is not whether peripheral colors are red or not red (or not blue), for they are certainly not red. But the question is whether they are identified with any of the definite normal colors, including the grays, and to this the answer seems to be "No."

If we regard peripheral vision as the most primitive surviving form, and this seems a reasonable assumption, then we have in its lack of definiteness a clue to the nature of qualitative evolution.[7]

A confirmation of this suggestion is found, surprisingly enough, in the mathematics of continuity. For just as the point cannot intelligibly be viewed as the actually existent element of space, nor the latter as a mere aggregate of points, so it is impossible to treat a qualitative member of a continuously varying series, like that of the colors, as literally a constituent of the continuum of color. Rather we are forced to construe the idea of a strictly single and absolutely definite color as an ideal limit of an abstractive set of more and more definite colors. In the

---

[7] For further evidence see Spearman, *The Nature of Intelligence*, chap. xiv.

midst of mathematical continuity the germ of qualitative evolution is thus sown, and an intelligible view of emergence provided for. According to this view, the emergent is not utterly incomparable to the pre-existing qualities, but is related to it as the more to the less determinate.

This conception, perhaps the most brilliant of those which we owe to the fertile brain of Charles Peirce,[8] is by no means free from prima facie difficulties. Peirce spoke as though the qualitative continuum in its primordial or non-generated aspect were not only without definite qualities but without definite dimensions—indeed, without any distinctions or contrasts of any kind. But in that case it nearly coincides with Aristotle's prime matter and is as unintelligible and useless for explanation. It is in accord with Peirce's own suggestions, however, to try to conceive the absolutely primordial factor as simply the general principle of divine love, with whatever contrasts, or at least germinal dimensions, may be involved in that conception.

If God contemplates any "eternal objects" with a contemplation that has had no birth and can have no death, then these objects need be no more than just the essence of love in its irreducible dimensions. The number of distinctions along any dimension which must thus be eternally contemplated appears arbitrary. Its self-enjoyment is the inexhaustible fountain of all that through its benevolence should ever come into being (into a share in this enjoyment). This is the light which may indeed be conceived always to have been shed upon the natures and the existences of things. The world may be conceived as the increasing specification of the theme "feeling of feeling."

---

[8] See his paper, "The Logic of Continuity," *Collected Papers*, Vol. VI; also my remarks in the *Philosophical Review*, XXXVIII, No. 3 (1929), 292-93.

# CHAPTER VII
# THE DIMENSIONS OF SENSATION

\*\*

*Given a number of dimensions of feeling, all possible varieties are obtainable by varying the intensities of the different elements.*

CHARLES S. PEIRCE

\*\*

### SECTION 32. COLOR

OF THE three Cartesian dimensions of the color solid, the only one which has been at all widely accepted as such is the vertical or black-white axis. Intermediaries between the two extremes of black and white have frequently been interpreted in terms of one common factor or variable, with positive, negative, and zero values. This variable is brightness. Yet, even in this favored instance, the dimensional analysis has not been the most popular one. A more usual view has been the atomistic conception of black and white as the simples of which the grays are compounds. The inadmissibility in principle of this view follows from considerations adduced in earlier chapters. Moreover, there is a further reason for denying the mixture hypothesis. What kind of mixture is it in which a reduction in the amount of one ingredient is *eo ipso* an increase in the amount of the other? When we speak of water as an ingredient of things in variable amounts, we know what we mean, because water is subject to these quantitative variations either in a pure state or while the amounts of other ingredients remain constant. But pure black and pure white have each but one degree, and the only way to decrease either is to adulterate it with the other. Thus there is no way of distinguishing between variations in the ratios of the alleged quantities and variations in the quantities themselves. Under such circumstances, what meaning does the quantitative idea retain?

A series of entities so related to two factors that approach toward the maximum of one of these two is *eo ipso* recession from the maximum of the other is not uncommon. Toward the right is *eo ipso* away from the left: stronger is *eo ipso* less weak; larger, *eo ipso* less small. In all such cases, however, the intermediate entities are not mixtures of the two extremes. In another type of series involving two opposite characters mixture does occur. For instance, income and expenditure are opposed, although one's financial state is a combination of the two. But here it is not true that an increase in income is of itself a decrease in outgo. Thus in every respect we see that the achromatic series classifies itself with series that do not involve mixture.[1]

It is instructive, furthermore, to note that the conception of gray as a black-white quasi-molecule has been attacked even from the atomistic standpoint. It occurred to Dimmick that the gray axis has certain features in common with the lines connecting complementary primaries: red-green, yellow-blue (waiving the question of the exact hues required for complementation). This analogy had, he found, escaped others because of an error in point of fact. Whereas, it had been thought, red-gray-green and yellow-gray-blue have as their common mid-points a color not in the least like, or involving either of, the extremes, the mid-point of black-gray-white is, on the contrary, nothing but a black-white in which both of the extremes are equally represented. Dimmick's subjects, however, could find in mid-gray no trace either of black or of white. Hence, concluded Dimmick, all three of the designated lines crossing in gray are of the same type, and should be used as the three co-ordinates of the color solid.[2]

It is always better precisely to invert a truth than to distort it at some wide, miscellaneous angle—for, in the former case, correction is easier. Now Dimmick's view seems such a precise inversion. There is a sense in which it is true that gray is neither black nor white, just as it is neither red nor green, yellow nor

[1] Cf. Pikler, *Schriften zur Anpassungstheorie*, I, 10–15.

[2] See F. L. Dimmick, "Note on the Series of Blacks, Grays, and Whites," *Psychological Review*, XXXII (1925), 334–36; "A Reinterpretation of the Color Pyramid," *ibid.*, XXXVI (1929), 83–90.

blue. But this sense is just the opposite of what Dimmick has in mind. His doctrine is that mid-gray, black, white, and the primaries are all simple factors, with all other colors their compound derivatives. But from his data he might have inferred the reverse of this. In a man of perfectly average or medium height there is no trace either of dwarfishness or of giantlikeness. We do not, however, infer that height is composed of three totally unlike qualities—tallness, shortness, and middle-sizedness. There is, rather, one quality, height, which has three critical values—extreme tallness, extreme shortness, and mean or normal height. Exactly so we may interpret the non-black and non-white character of mid-gray. If white is extreme brilliance, black, extreme lack of brilliance, then obviously in mid-gray there is no trace whatever of either. For there can be nothing extreme, whether of abundance or of deficiency, in the absolute mean of brilliance. On the other hand, Dimmick may be perfectly right in saying that the relations of mid-gray to the complementary chromas are formally similar to its relations to black and white. For there may be other variables besides brilliance which have midvalues in mean gray; and the extreme values of these other variables may constitute the primary chromas, as the extremes of brilliance constitute black and white. The utility of Dimmick's observations is that they show the complete inadequacy of the usual grounds for denying such common variables to complementary pairs. We do not seem to see anything redlike or greenlike in gray; hence it does not occur to us that red-green-gray can be different values of one variable. We do most of us see something blacklike and whitelike in gray; hence the notion of a common factor of brilliance easily arises. But it is now clear that whether or not the extremes are seen in the mean depends on the sense in which they are conceived, and that the inability of most of us to see the redlikeness of gray may derive from the same causes as Dimmick's inability to elicit the black-white character of mid-gray. What needs explanation is only the more common occurrence of the former inability. The explanation is not difficult. The one variable we must always be conscious of as such in vision is brightness. The achromatic series is the only one which visual abnormalities cannot obliterate while vision itself remains. The reason is that degrees of brilliance are essentially degrees of strength of visual stimulation (per unit of area, distinguishable as such), and while we are conscious of stimulation at all, we cannot but be affected by sufficiently marked differences in the strength of the stimulus.

We have now arrived at another difficulty in the interpretation of gray, black, and white. Is black the zero of visual intensity? Can there not be an intense black? And is not black a positive sensation rather than the absence of sensation? The answer is that the lack of something may, precisely as a lack, be definitely and so, if you will, positively apprehended. Just so is black the positive apprehension of the complete lack of brightness, of visual intensity. Back of our heads we see nothing; but we do not definitely apprehend this failure of vision as such; hence it is not black for us. But where we expect to see and do not, there we "see" black. And the quality of black is just the quality of failure, of sheer denial of life and of joy or sorrow, the quality of death. Black is not the color of mourning, in some nations, because of associations, nor yet because it is a sad color, but because it is the sheer evil of non-being (the only absolute evil, in spite of Schopenhauer). No color is objectively ugly save this one, which is employed in art only as a foil to enable us to realize to the full the true positivity of the remaining colors. It is good only as the good life does not consist in the unconsciousness of evil.

Of course, darkness can be restful and welcome. But then it is not definitely apprehended as such and is not black, but gray or brown or violet. And if a black dress can be enjoyed, it is because the face seen with the dress, or the glints of light here and there, are not black; nor can black be seen at all unrelieved by something more rewarding. For a person to be able to choose black as a favorite color, he must be much more than "half in love with easeful death"—in fact, such choice is scarcely a sincere possibility.

Thus in this crucial instance we see at once the unity of mind and its contents, and the roughly describable character of sensory quality. The whole nature of life as a seeking of values, plotted against a background of the possible destruction of these values, is concentrated in an intense black, the keen vision of the abhorrent loss, at a certain point, of all intensity. The black-white contrast is not something absolutely unique and peculiar to vision but only an especially distinct form of a general contrast that pervades all experience. The special distinctness characterizing the visual form is readily explained. The explanation is furnished by a writer who was quite innocent of such a doctrine as the one just expounded. Mrs. Ladd-Franklin points to the unique spatial definiteness and completeness of visual experience, its tendency to form a plenum, as the reason for the fact that non-stimulation of a part of the retina gives a definite sensation.[3] Pikler emphasizes the same consideration, but adds to it the further conceptions necessary to explain why this sensation should have the character which it has, rather than, say, the character of the sensation in fact produced by positive monochromatic stimuli, or by white light. Why do we not see physical darkness as green or yellow or white? To this question orthodox psychology has no answer except a veto upon the question. All the while the true answer is missed only because it is so obvious and so close to us. We simply could not have felt about the absence of light in a white or yellow or green fashion. The qualities of these colors are not appropriate to the disappointment of the desire to see. Black is thus appropriate.[4]

If the reader asks for the evidence upon which these statements are made, the answer of course is "in one word, experience." Gloom and evil and annihilation are directly intuited in black, never joy and success and fulness of life. Then there is the indirect evidence from aesthetic practice, etc., which of course raises interpretational problems involving the rôle of associations and other supersensory factors.

The feature of the chromatic visual qualities which more than any other seems to have impressed the earliest inquirers is the

---

[3] C. Ladd-Franklin, *Colour and Colour Theories* (New York, 1929), pp. 244 f.
[4] Pikler, *op. cit.*, I, 1-33.

fact that hue, although a dimension of variation distinct from brightness, is nevertheless not at right angles to the latter dimension (as our textbooks rather carelessly represent it), but slants sharply, so that among the fully saturated colors yellow is approximately the brightest, violet is the darkest, and red and green are about equally bright. Aristotle, Goethe, and Pikler have rightly insisted that its ability to explain this fact is one of the principal tests of the validity of any theory of color. The failure of Hering's attempt to furnish such an explanation is generally conceded. But the other best-known theories succeed no better in this respect. Indeed, it is a characteristic of most modern theories to ignore the problem, to furnish explanations of red, yellow, green, and blue which would be equally relevant if it were not a fact that a saturated blue is always less bright than a saturated yellow.

The first thing we may infer from the differential relations of colors to brightness is a partial explanation of the "primacy" of certain colors—those often called simple—and the secondary character of the others. It seems intelligible that orange and yellow-green, for example, should not have been felt as fundamental points in the color series, for the natural procedure was to group together all yellowish colors, from orange to yellow-green, as the conspicuously bright colors, the colors of sunlight, in contrast to the blues and purples, which are the dull or shadow colors. (Consider Homer's phrase, the "wine-dark sea.") As for the reds and greens, they would naturally be left as transition hues, colors neither very dark nor very bright, and yet inevitably distinguished from each other as red from green or vice versa, in spite of the agreement in respect to brightness, because of their sharp contrast in another respect (to be discussed presently). Thus four colors would inevitably appear as fundamental: the brightest, yellow; the dullest, blue; and the two unmistakably different colors of neutral brightness, red and green. So far no need whatsoever arises to posit any peculiar simplicity as the ground for primacy.

The chief defect of this account lies in the fact that the blue which seems to be felt as primary is not the dullest blue, the latter being characterized as a slightly reddish-blue, i.e., violet. This certainly shows that the explanation so far proposed is not the whole truth, though it by no means eliminates it as representing a very real part of the truth. The complete explanation may be complicated. In the first place, the violet which we see is, owing to subjective impurities introduced by the eye, not a "true" or "pure" violet, but contains always a mixture of longer wave-lengths.[5] Perhaps this is the reason why violet appears a dependent rather than a fundamental color. The hypothetical true violet might make blue appear as a green-violet. Yet this introduction of physiological considerations is of questionable relevance, since the subject under discussion is the phenomenal colors in their directly given relationships, not in relation to the physical character of stimuli. But even in purely phenomenal terms there is reason to consider the violet we experience as a somewhat desaturated color, and this weakens its capacity to appear as a critical turning-point in the color scale. The fact that olive-green, also an unsaturated color, should seem at once reddish, yellowish, and greenish, whereas in full saturation yellow-green seems free of red, shows that the reddishness of actual violet does not disprove the primacy of real or pure violet. The fact that apparently no one can experience the latter proves nothing at all against this assumption—does not in the least show that if the eye had permitted pure violet stimulation, undisturbed by fluorescence, we should not have seen blue as a green-violet.

A further factor which might account for a displacement of the dull primary is the relative frequency of blue in nature as compared to that of violet and purple. It is difficult to assess the weight to be accorded to such widely differing influences. But clearly the first essential is to recognize the complexity of the problem, instead of adopting our impressions of primacy as infallible evidences of the exact qualitative situation. When so many causes of error can be imagined (we shall mention others presently), it would be rather surprising if no error had occurred.

The conception of the primaries as critical points of bright-

[5] See L. T. Troland, *Sensation*, par. 323.

ness obviously requires supplementation. It is clear that the difference between chromas cannot be one of brightness alone; for then saturated and unsaturated colors would be indistinguishable. Yellow is not characterized merely as a bright color, nor red merely as one of medium brightness. Three dimensions cannot be conjured out of one.

It is a general impression that yellow is not simply a bright—i.e., intense—color, but that it has a more specific quality which is somehow comparable to a feeling of joy, and that blue, and still more violet, has an opposite character which relates it to melancholy. Whatever, in more precise terms, these characters are, it is in them that we must seek the second of the three dimensions of color variation.

The contrast of red and green has by no means appeared to men and women in general as ineffable. At least two descriptive adjectives are commonly applied to it: "activity," with its correlate, passivity; and "warmth," with its opposite, coolness. Red light-rays stimulate, excite, and suggest heat; green rays quiet, and suggest cold. Red is violent, green is gentle; red seems also to advance toward the spectator, creating a slight illusion of greater nearness than the other color where both are in fact the same distance away. The curious thing is that although all of these characterizations occur in reds and greens of equal brightness, there seems to be a closer relationship between the red characteristics and those of bright colors, or between the green and those of dark colors, than between red and dark, or green and bright, color qualities. Thus bright colors as well as red ones tend to advance, and to appear active and warm; dull, as well as green, colors to recede and to impress one as cold. And it must be confessed that the maximum of warmth is as often as not thought to lie at yellow rather than red, and of cold at blue or even violet rather than green. In so far as this occurs, doubt must arise concerning the legitimacy of seeing in warmth the third color dimension. There is also the question whether or not warm refers to the same qualitative aspect as active, aggressive, advancing. All three may be related yet distinct, and their maxima may lie at different though perhaps neighboring points.

In spite of these difficulties, it is fairly demonstrable that the descriptive adjectives in question do indicate the nature of the red-green rather than the yellow-violet contrast. For while it is true that yellow is often called the warmest color, it is also true that red, and never by any accident green, is so regarded; and while blue, or even violet, is often called the cold maximum, never by any chance do we find red thus characterized. Again, the slightest inclination of yellow toward green has a cooling effect totally unmatched by that of a slight redlikeness of yellow. Indeed is not a yellow-orange felt as warmer than yellow? And all these remarks hold of active-passive characterizations. Another piece of evidence against the assumption that the thermal contrast coincides with that between yellow and blue is that of actual thermal sensations. It is a very well-attested fact that cold is brighter than warm—indicating the very opposite from a violet affinity for cold. To be sure this fact remains a paradox even if we locate cold at green, but a much less acute one than if we locate it at a still duller color.

The evidence for the reality of an activity-passivity character in red-green includes physiological tests[6] and statistical, experimental ones, as well as the unanimous opinion of artists and practical workers in color. As a working hypothesis, its legitimacy is abundantly established. But the difficulties which the hypothesis must meet include, besides those already mentioned, numerous more detailed uncertainties or apparent discrepancies. For instance, even if red is the most active color, it does not appear that this red is the non-spectral hue which the psychologists select as "pure" or standard red. Rather it is spectral scarlet which would probably be chosen as the warmth maximum. Similarly, the coldest green is not pure but bluish green, sea-green, that which by the test of complementation lies opposite scarlet. But if this is true, then we have to explain away the seeming primacy or purity of so-called pure red and green, just as we had formerly to explain away the seeming primacy of

---

[6] See K. Goldstein and O. Rosenthal, "Zum Problem der Wirkung der Farben auf den Organismus," *Archives suisses de neurologie et de psychiatrie*, XXVI (1930), 3-26. For a summary of this work see *Psychological Abstracts*, VI (1932), 2084.

blue. Thus instead of accounting for the primaries, we appear to be engaged in denying them. And yet, to locate the real primaries at a point somewhat near to but not coincident with the points designated by ordinary impressions is not necessarily an illegitimate procedure, unless absolute accuracy is to be expected of such impressions. Supposing scarlet to be the true critical point concerned in red, it is arguable that an illusory critical point—in a certain sense a real one—would occur in the red-purples; and, similarly, accepting blue-green as the truly characteristic green, reasons can be given for the impression that a color really yellow-green is pure green.

Scarlet, we are told, is impure red; for it is possible to detect a slight yellowlikeness in this color. In non-spectral red this yellow affinity vanishes without giving place to an opposite or blue-suggesting impurity. But it is a first principle of dimensional qualitative analysis that every color has resemblance to every other, so that if we define pure red as a totally unyellowlike color, this unyellowlikeness requires careful qualification. Yellow is one maximum of a factor which is at a neutral midvalue (but not at an opposite maximum) in red. Thus red is unyellowlike in just the sense in which mid-gray is neither black nor white. Hence, just as it is possible to see a white affinity in a mid-gray, so it should be possible to see a suggestion of yellow in pure red. But should it not also be possible to see a similar relation between pure red and violet, to see scarlet as a variation of violet as well as of yellow? It should, no doubt, be possible, and I dare say it is so, but it need not, for all that, be equally easy. For yellow is a bright, that is to say an intense or strong, color; and consequently it tends to dominate its weaker opposite and to give really pure red a pseudo-contamination with yellow, while violet is relatively unable to effect such contamination. Weak violet retreats before yellow, dragging red with it to purple.

To test this reasoning, let us apply it to the opposite side of the color circle, the green sector. At once we confront a difficulty. If yellow tends to dominate, why should not apparent green also retreat, like apparent red, toward violet? But we have assumed that the true green is sea-green, and hence that apparent green is really yellow-green. Shall we *ad hoc* renounce the explanation which proved so convenient for red? Well, there is this at least to be said. Apparent green is not, it seems to me, judged pure primarily on account of its freedom from yellow. The greatest danger of confusion is not between green and yellow, but between green and blue, just as it is far easier to confuse what is called orange than what is called purple with red. A green may be nearly pure and still strongly suggest blue, while a green must be far indeed toward yellow to be in any danger of confusion with that color. But to say this is only to state the problem over again. Why are these things so? The answer may lie in the fact, already commented upon, that apparent blue is really a green-violet, i.e., has suffered displacement toward green. Consequently green itself is compelled, to save itself from blue contamination, to flee toward yellow, until a point is reached where the danger from that color equals the danger from blue. Because of the greater strength of the former color, the resulting locus of green will be a little nearer to apparent blue than to yellow.

The hypothetical displacements of blue, red, and green may also be summarized as follows. There are two strong colors, yellow and red. In some curious way the strength of one is different in nature and not merely in degree from that of the other. There results a natural tendency to orient color description about these two, but most of all about yellow, the brightest color. Now, as the most striking differences are those which are greatest in degree, the color which will be emphasized along with red and yellow is that one which is equally unlike both. This color is blue. Red, yellow, and blue approximately trisect the color system. In no color is it harder to detect likeness to either red or yellow than in blue. Thus, granting that red and yellow have been selected as primaries, blue is bound to appear fundamental also. There remain the three intermediaries of red, yellow, and blue, i.e., orange, green, and purple. Orange can hardly escape assimilation to red and yellow, the two most vigorous of colors. Purple betrays red and blue, and is both a dull and, in nature, a rare, inconspicuous hue. Green can, in spite of numerous denials, be seen as a yellow-blue. Brentano, probably most artists, and many other persons have asserted such a perception, and the contention that they have merely fallen here into the stimulus error, i.e., confused their knowledge of pigment-mixing with directly perceived relationships, is a convenient rebuttal but has nothing evidential about it. But green is the commonest of all colors in nature, and is a brighter color than purple; so it resists such assimilation better than the latter.

So far we have ventured to tamper, by way of experiment, with every primary save yellow. But if we think of this as the brightest color, there is evidence that here, too, apparent and real purity fail to coincide. For the yellow whose luminosity is by most tests shown as maximum is not quite the same as that adjudged pure, but rather a slightly lemon hue, buttercup yellow. This is a slightly colder color than apparent yellow, and the latter is really slightly reddish. It appears that yellow is less sensitive to contamination from red than vice versa, and also less than it is to contamination from green. The former circumstance we may ascribe to the brightness superiority of yellow to red, the latter to the curious hostility that obtains between yellow and green as compared to the equally paradoxical congruence between yellow and red. Red, like yellow, is strong, even though not in the same sense. Green is in no sense particularly strong or striking.

From Goethe to Pikler dimensional theorists have recognized this affinity of red to the bright and of green to the dark colors, in spite of the fact that red is not bright and green is not dark. Aesthetically, red and black form a much more dynamical contrast than a green of the same brightness and black. The Chinese use of scarlet-and-black combinations is not, I think, paralleled by any similar use of black and a green of the same brilliance as Chinese red. That dynamical opposition is not the same as merely wide difference is perhaps also shown by the fact that black letters against a yellow background have been found to possess greater visibility than black letters against a white background, although the mere difference (number of just noticeable differences) between the first pair of colors is probably not greater.

Our four real primaries, how legitimately determined only further study can show, are then: scarlet (warmth-activity), buttercup yellow (brightness and joyousness), sea-green (cold-passivity), violet (dulness and sorrowfulness). If we call the scarlet-green factor $W$ (for warmth) and the yellow-violet $H$ (for happiness, joyousness), then red may be defined as $W_{+1} H_0$ (warmth positive, joyousness neutral); yellow as $W_0 H_{+1}$ (warmth neutral, joyousness positive); green as $W_{-1} H_0$ (warmth negative, joyousness neutral); violet as $W_0 H_{-1}$ (warmth neutral, joyousness negative). Intermediate colors can be indicated by decimals, thus: $H_{+.7} W_{+.7}$, or $\frac{7}{10}$ happy and $\frac{7}{10}$ warm, i.e., an orange approximately halfway between scarlet and buttercup; or $H_{+.7} W_{-.7}$, $\frac{7}{10}$ happy and $\frac{7}{10}$ cold, yellow-green.

The meaning of primacy in this system is clearly seen. Obviously, $H_{+.7} W_{-.7}$ is an intermediary between $H_0 W_{-1}$ and $H_{+1} W_0$, since it possesses in moderate degree the factor maximally present in the one and that similarly present in the other. On the other hand, if we consider $H_{+.7} W_{+.7}$ and $H_{+.7} W_{-.7}$, the characteristic of each will seem to be lost in the intermediary $H_{+1} W_0$. Orange loses its positive warmth, and yellow-green its coldness. What remains of each is only the $H_{+.7}$, which is but a lesser degree of the $H_{+1}$, the distinctive property of yellow. Naturally, then, we feel that what connects yellow to orange and yellow-green is just yellowishness, whereas we feel that orange is connected to red by reddishness and to yellow by yellowishness, i.e., we think of orange as compounded of its neighbors, yellow as simple. All combining of colors separated by a primary results in neutralization of at least one variable by virtue of opposite signs. It involves thus the principle of complementation, but complementary relationships in the pregnant or ordinary sense result when two combined colors separated by a primary are themselves neutral with respect to one variable (this occurs only with colors themselves primary) or when they have opposite signs and equal values in terms of both variables. Comple-

## PLATE II

### Dimensions of Color

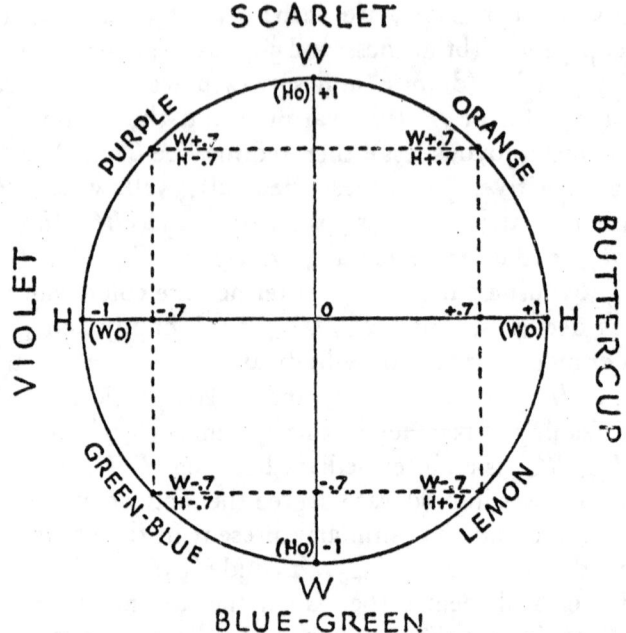

The circle should in reality be flattened in some parts, since saturation is not uniform. Still other irregularities may be involved.

The four principal secondary colors or half-way points between primaries lie, for geometrical reasons, at c.±.7 rather than ±.5 or the arithmetical mean values.

The problem of color harmony will be seen to be more complex than was recognized in section 22. For instance, secondary colors a quarter-circle apart will not, like primary colors so separated, suffer from lack of resemblance, but from a lack of balance between positive and negative with respect to the common property (+.7 or −.7). There will be an unsatisfied demand for contrast, for values of opposite sign, whereas the zero or neutral factor uniting complementary primaries is more self-sufficient. Complementary secondaries appear to have nothing in common; but they share in a common lack of neutrality values: a common degree, though opposite sign, of eccentricity from the mean.

mentary neutralization is merely a limiting case of all intermediation which crosses an axis of the color system. It requires no special explanation whatsoever.

A further advantage of this system over the traditional one of simple qualities is that the triadic law of color mixture is deducible from it, as it certainly is not from the traditional system. From the notion of four simple atoms of quality and their molecular combinations, or from the notion of simples corresponding to all possible colors, the two forms taken by the traditional theory, no one could possibly guess, what is of course the fact, that all colors can be produced by combinations of three, and not less than three, stimuli. But from the notion of four critical turning-points in a continuum of similarities generated by a pair of co-ordinates, this possibility does follow and is simply the geometrical truism that three points and their intermediates are sufficient to constitute a self-returning line, or that three points are required and are sufficient to determine a plane.[7] This geometrical truth is also an intuitive one in the application to color. For instance, all colors besides red, yellow, and blue, can be seen as either red-yellows, yellow-blues (greens), or red-blues. Or again, though less easily, all colors in addition to orange, lemon, and purple can be seen as orange-lemon (a rather tan-yellow), lemon-purple (a grayed blue or green), or purple-orange (brownish red). The difficulty of this second instance is due to the pervasiveness of partial neutralization, owing to the non-primary colors chosen.

In order to save the simplicity doctrine and yet account for the triadic law, Brentano denied the primacy of green and proposed red, yellow, and blue as the only primaries. But since the law can be deduced from the assumption of four non-simple primaries, the notion of simplicity, which leaves inexplicable many other facts likewise deducible from the alternative notion, is hardly helped by this proposal.

Another advantage of the system above outlined is that it divides the circle of hues into more nearly equal steps between

---

[7] The three-process theory of vision is not necessarily invalidated by this reasoning. But the alleged evidence for it requires re-examination.

primaries. The accepted green and blue are crowded close to each other and to yellow, and far away from red, which is also very far from yellow.[8] By shifting red to scarlet, yellow less sharply to buttercup, green again sharply to blue-green, blue to something like violet, the spacing can be made more equal, and at the same time complementation between red and green, yellow and its opposite primary, preserved.

Finally, in the dimensions of the color solid, so conceived, we can perhaps discern the modes of variation which we have denoted the ultimate dimensions of mind. Activity-passivity, joy-sorrow, and intensity-faintness are the three qualitative variables of experience as a social-affective continuum. To them correspond red-green, yellow-violet, white-black. The sensory status as such resides in the objectification, i.e., the position on the structural dimension of depth or social otherness. The specifically visual character lies in the relation to the eye, in the exceptionally exact value of the cross-dimensional spatial order, and in certain minor peculiarities involving the same fundamental social variables. Thus all the main features of color are susceptible of at least rough or vague definition in terms that are intelligible quite apart from color experience, e.g., to one born blind. So far from an established truth is the dogma that a color is an ineffable quality!

A final question is this: Why, among colors, is yellow the brightest, violet the dullest, while red and green are about equally bright? In terms of our social-affective variables, the following answer suggests itself: Red and green express states of social unbalance; for in the one the object dominates, tyrannizes over, the subject, and in the other the object submits, recedes, gives way to the subject. But the ideal relation is neither of these, but rather one of harmony, balance, reciprocity. It seems reasonable to suppose that such a balanced relation can occur at a higher intensity than either form of the unbalanced. In the upper ranges of strength such harmony may naturally be joyous, i.e., yellow, in the lower, melancholy, i.e., violet. However, there is also a balance between joy and sorrow, and

[8] Cf. Troland, *op. cit.*, pp. 144-45.

this will be the most complete single quality of all and will be able to occur at a higher intensity than any other, i.e., white. In similar fashion we can deal with the fact that violet is the dullest of primaries, while black is duller than any chroma. For unbalance in the social relation cannot be extreme—red or green—unless one of the two aspects of the relation is present in considerable strength, whereas harmony can be at any intensity above zero. And, finally, the contrast between joy and sorrow cannot be marked where the zero of intensity is approached, so that social balance to be melancholy—violet—must be well above black in brightness. Black is balance between joy and sorrow at the vanishing-point of non-being; white is the same at the maximum of endurable intensity.

### SECTION 33. SOUND

It is a notable peculiarity of hearing that an apparently single dimension, that of pitch, should produce combination effects of a totally different type from any to be met with elsewhere in a uni-dimensional series. For instance, the grays may be combined at will without producing anything similar to octave relationships in music; whereas, when the other dimensions of color variation are employed, harmonic relations comparable, to a certain extent at least, to the musical may be obtained. The explanation is usually seen in the force of association or custom. For physical reasons we are used to certain tonal combinations, those most frequently involved in tone-overtone complexes, hence the effects of smoothness and fusion characterizing these combinations, and also the contrary effects of the more unusual intervals. Experiments showing the gain in acceptability of discords through repetition bear this out.

This explanation almost certainly involves a truth, but the interpretation of this truth is subject to important qualifications. First, granting that constant conjunction in experience is the cause of octave relationships, it by no means follows that these relationships consist simply in the sense of familiarity or smoothness produced by this conjunction. For the causes of aesthetic experience, as of any other kind, are one set of entities, its constituent, phenomenal characters quite another. Now if there are any universal or necessary constituents of aesthetic experience, they are likenesses and differences appreciable as such. If we do not know this, we know practically nothing in aesthetics. Since the outstanding characteristic of octave relationships is their periodicity, the immediate inference to be drawn is that their likenesses and differences are similarly periodic. The strength of this inference is quite independent of the question of causes. Aesthetic experience is not the mere undergoing of an effect; it is the direct intuition of relationships embodied in what is immediately presented. The production of this immediate content is another matter. Supposing constant conjunction to be the ultimate cause, the effect of harmony is one which there is reason to believe could only be produced if the cause acts by modifying the qualitative content so as to render its parts alike and different in the required manner.[9] More explicitly put, the inference from musical experience is that more than one dimension of qualitative variation is involved in the tonal scale, that the pure tones ascend not in the order of a straight line but, say, in that of a spiral, with a periodic return to the same points in the dimensions additional to that of pitch height.

Similar remarks obviously apply to explanations of harmony through ratios of wave-lengths. The explanation is persuasive, only it leaves the problem of description, of analysis of the presented aesthetic design, quite untouched. I do not deny that sound waves as such are intuited; but I am pointing out that if they are, it is with the utmost faintness or unclearness, so that introspection is almost completely powerless to detect them as separate items in consciousness. What follows is not that these items are not given, not real constituents of the phenomena, but that they are far indeed from being among the most prominent of such constituents, and that they are not the major descriptive features to be stressed in attempting to trace the aesthetic design. And we are asking: "What are those features?"

[9] Pikler, whose theory of consonance is rather different from the one I am suggesting, insists that "consonance is perception of similarity, sameness." He differs only in the specification of the nature of the similarities (*op. cit.*, II, 31).

The insufficiency of the causal account is also shown in the fact that it does not do justice to the difference between fusion and consonance. The most readily fused pairs are the octaves, but there are several much richer intervals than these. And then, is the impression of musical chords at all like that to be expected from a fusion of grays, of a one-dimensional series? The question, however, may be objected to on the ground that in vision fusion in this sense does not occur. Only sounds possess timbre—that is to say, a Gestalt quality which, although a unitary thing, can nevertheless be analyzed into simpler constituents in a manner unduplicated in vision. But this difference is easily exaggerated. If very small but not wholly indistinguishable patches of different colors are juxtaposed, the effect is neither that of a single homogeneous color nor yet that of clearly distinguishable separate colors, but of a more or less complete blend of color tones.[10] The result well deserves the name of visual timbre, and the systematic use of such timbre in painting is the technical innovation of the impressionists. The only truth in the denial of visual timbre is one of degree; and it lies in the vastly superior distinctness of spatialization of colors as compared to sounds, the result of which is that sound components are almost always partially confused together to a degree ordinarily either greatly exceeded (as in pigment mixtures, where the separate color areas cannot as such be introspected at all) or far from equaled (as in most juxtaposed color patches of appreciable size) by color components.

The visual analogy directs our attention to an important feature of timbre, which is that in proportion as the distinctness of the constituents recedes, the Gestalt quality of the complex approaches in character the simple quality produced by a homogeneous stimulus. Contiguous specks of yellow and blue pigment produce simply green, unless the specks are of barely discernible magnitude, when the effect is not exactly that of green nor yet very different from it. In audition there are almost if not quite innumerable degrees of this transition; but it remains true that just in so far as the constituents as such are blurred, the

[10] See Franz Brentano, *Untersuchungen zur Sinnespsychologie*, p. 89.

over-all quality approaches simplicity. The dogma that timbre is absolutely peculiar to sounds means, in last analysis, the denial that the principle just enunciated holds of them. But there seems no reason to except audition from the principle that an over-all or complex quality is given as different from a simple quality only just in so far as the complex as such is really given. The principle seems self-evident, and I know of no fact with which it conflicts. The consequence is that the problem of auditory quality is complicated by the presence of timbre only in so far as separate constituents become prominent, apart from which prominence the qualities of timbre need not be very different from the qualities which, so far as simplicity is concerned, might be those of pure tones. It follows that the number of dimensions of unitary qualities of audition need not have the magnitude suggested by the endlessness of overtone possibilities.

If the series of pure tones is multi-dimensional and periodic, spiral-like, then there exists among the pure tones no series corresponding to the line of neutral grays. The center of the spiral of pure tones is hollow. But to this extent hearing is precisely like vision. In both senses homogeneous stimuli generally produce saturated sensations. The difference is that in vision heterogeneous stimuli produce unsaturated sensations, provided these stimuli are separated by a complementary interval, i.e., provided their normal sensations are approximately opposite on the hue circle; whereas in hearing, according to Ohm's law of analysis, instead of complementary cancellation of chroma, complementary harmony is all that can result from two stimuli which are opposite each other on the octave spiral circle. Nevertheless, auditory gray is a deducible possibility under certain conditions, and under those conditions it appears to be a fact. It is known that Ohm's law is largely suspended if a band of neighboring frequencies occur simultaneously, for "when the basilary apparatus .... is excited by two closely similar frequencies of about equal intensities,"[11] an intermediate tone is experienced which seems to indicate that there is "an intermediate section of the membrane which is vibrating at both of the

[11] Troland, *op. cit.*, p. 252.

given frequencies at once," so that there is "a partial failure of analysis." Now suppose that a band of frequencies which are thus fused together into a "compromise" frequency does not cover more than a quarter or a sixth of an octave. The compromise will possess some tonal saturation, just as various hues of orange ranging from a very red to a very yellow hue fuse together into one recognizable though somewhat desaturated orange. But if the band covers a third or nearly one-half an octave, its extremes are in nearly the complementary relationship, which, given the suspension of analysis, implies, if the compromise effect concerns the octave quality as well as the brightness of the extremes, as in vision it affects both hue and brightness, a more or less complete neutralization of octave quality, i.e., auditory gray. Now these conditions are often realized, and the resulting experience is known as vowel quality. Where the spread of the unanalyzed frequencies is less than four halftones, the result is, as the foregoing deduction implies, a musical tone with slight vowel quality;[12] where it is more than a semi-octave, the result is a vowel with a noise character.[13]

The conclusion is that, as Jaensch has forcibly argued, the vowels are the "qualities of noises," in so far as noises have definite simple characters, and that these qualities of noises are desaturated or mere brightnesses, i.e., auditory grays, in which, however, the exact degree of brightness is more or less indeterminate, owing to the incompleteness of the suppression of analysis in the auditory case. This blurring of the shade of pitch brightness increases with the spread of the frequencies so that it is greatest with non-vocalic noises, or those which cover considerably more than the range necessary for complementation. Those covering less than this range become more and more similar to pure musical tones, but with some remnant of vowel quality or desaturation until practically homogeneous stimuli are reached. Thus if we had never experienced vowels we could have deduced from other features of auditory experi-

[12] Jaensch, *Untersuchungen über Grundfragen der Akustik und Tonpsychologie*, pp. 9-11 (Kurve III).

[13] *Ibid.* (Kurve IV).

ence that such sensations would probably occur.[14] That they cover five octaves is not surprising since it is only over some such range that octave quality is pronounced and since above or below this range desaturation would occur without complementation, and would thus lack the blurring of brightness characteristic of auditory as distinct from visual gray, besides suggesting something analogous to black and white, rather than to gray as the intermediate brightness experience, leaving out of account the evidence (discussed in sec. 6B) that very high pitches do not advance "upward" so much as they suffer displacement in a topographical rather than qualitative scheme. Even the validity of Ohm's law, as well as the restrictions to this validity, are deducible from phenomenal characteristics of sound. For analysis presupposes spatial or temporal separation, and fusion spatio-temporal overlapping; so that the relative vagueness of auditory spatialization implies that various degrees of fusion are possible, whereas the precision of visual localization means that separate colors will be much more definitely or absolutely separate than sounds. Thus our description of the characters of auditory phenomena apart from vowels and noises enables us to deduce the main characters of the latter, thus verifying a virtual prediction derived from the description, since the latter was not adopted with the vowels or noises in mind.

If a certain mode of combination of pure tones results in partial or complete loss of saturation, it is possible that another type of combination would have the opposite result of increasing saturation. Several reasons, indeed, incline us to consider the saturation of pure tones as less than maximal. If it were maximal, it could scarcely have been so largely overlooked as to cause the notion of a merely one-dimensional tonal series to acquire the currency which, in fact, it has acquired. Furthermore, if, as the notion of octave quality requires, the same tone color is to be repeated at different pitch-brightness levels, and

[14] The actual production of speech vowels is, however, a more complicated and varied process than the foregoing discussion suggests. See Richard Paget, *Human Speech* (London, 1930), chaps. iii-v; and P. Kucharski, in *Nature*, November 11, 1933, p. 752.

if, as we seem to learn from vision, maximal saturation is possible at but one brightness, then but one of the repetitions at most can represent full saturation. Even this one instance, however, involves a difficulty. If tone color is to vary in more than one dimension, there must be one or more of its dimensions which is at right angles to the brightness axis; that is, there must be two color qualities which are opposite to each other, as are red and green, for example, but which are not, in full saturation, very different in brightness. Such qualities could not occur in a spiral of octave-related pitches in which all tones widely different in quality must also be widely different in brightness. Now the assumption of octave quality derives a considerable portion of its significance from implications depending on its being not less than two-dimensional. So we must conclude that the saturation of pure tones in contrast to noises admits of degrees, and that the maximal degrees which actually occur may not be found among the pure tones. This means that they are to be sought among the tonal combinations other than noises. There is no a priori reason, indeed, why a mode of tonal synthesis should not occur in which the qualities of the constituents should receive added emphasis by virtue of their union in this synthesis. The effects of color contrast are worth recalling in this connection.

In one respect the analogy between colors and tones appears complete. The darkest and the brightest colors, the lowest and the highest tones, are unsaturated. It is recognized that, at extremes of high and low, tones lose their musical character, i.e., their octave quality or tone color, not merely their pitch definiteness. (For a possible reason for this see pp. 224–25.)

The feeling that sounds are not comparable to colors is partly due to our habit of thinking chiefly, in this connection, of "surface" colors. If "light" colors, "shine," and atmospheric or "depth" colors, are taken into account, together with the subjective or pre-sensational qualities discussed in section 17, it will be more readily seen that the characteristic difference between sound and color, as well as that between both and the more subjunctive aspects of experience, admits of degrees.

There is a very particular physiological ground for the seemingly curious assumption that pure tones should vary always in more than one dimension at once. This is that they are never really pure tones, owing to the "subjective overtones" produced in the ear mechanism. "Our conception of a pure tone," says Troland, "must . . . . be adulterated with that of its harmonics, as 'subjectively' generated."[15] This, as Troland points out, removes the difficulty previously found in the Helmholtz theory of tonal fusion, and at the same time provides a basis for the phenomena of octave periodicity. Musically related tones have common constituents physiologically, which means not so much that they have common constituents psychologically—for they may not be given with any psychological complexity which is sufficiently clear cut to count—but it does suggest that they will have psychological resemblance. Hence the physiological impurity of even the purest tones implies that, since the change from pitch to pitch will affect the relative strengths of the subjective overtones, the change in tonal quality will be in more than one dimension, and will exhibit octave relationships. Also the merely partial saturation of pure tones in comparison to certain timbres may be explained, inasmuch as the effect of the higher notes in the latter would be to reinforce the overtone elements of the lower notes, thus emphasizing the factors entering into the octave quality of the lower notes. This, however, is only a suggestion. Quite different aspects of the auditory mechanism may be of equal or greater significance in the production of octave quality.

Can anyone persuade himself that the rich and motley arrays of tone color enjoyed in music could arise from the compounding of qualities restricted to the meager allowance of one dimension of qualitative variation?[16] The theory of uni-dimensional tonal quality is strangely unsuggestive, indeed, of any of the main facts of musical experience save one—the fact that pure tones

---

[15] *Op. cit.*, p. 253.

[16] Brentano (*op. cit.*, p. 102) declares: "No one will admit that a Beethoven symphony is painted all in gray." Brentano's conclusion is in some respects similar to the one presented in this section.

of the s? pitch and volume (and loudness, if that is not determined by the two former attributes) are always of the same quality. But a spiral fits this fact quite as well as does a straight line, the linearity, not the dimensional number alone, being relevant. The uni-dimensionalists reduce all music to etching in black and white, and attempt to conceal the unplausibility of their assumption by pretending that timbre is a uniquely auditory phenomenon whereby saturation springs out of neutrality; whereas in fact timbre in color is not wanting precisely upon condition that we do not limit our consideration to achromatic colors—colors in one dimension only. The impressionists, who were the most pronounced exploiters of visual timbre, were painters who also emphasized chroma.

Accepting the spiral hypothesis, we reach the heart of the problem of sound in the question: How are the dimensions additional to pitch brightness—though, in pure tones, not variable independently of variations in that dimension—to be described? Once more, we may consult speech usages for suggestions, though not for proofs, and we find that sound-descriptive adjectives are not uncommon. Tones are called warm, cold, joyous, etc. We have seen that warm colors are the reddish, cool colors the blue-greenish. There is a tendency for the warm colors to be somewhat brighter than the cool, but neither warm nor cold extreme seems to coincide with that of light or dark. All this suggests that the most pronouncedly warm and cold tones will be those of moderate pitch, with the warmest perhaps somewhat higher. We must, however, not overlook the fact that thermal warm is duller than thermal cold. My own experience, at any rate, is that the most pronounced effect of warmth is in certain relatively low tones of stringed instruments, and in certain higher notes of the trumpet. The latter tones suggest scarlet, as long ago remarked; the former suggest a warm red-violet. This is consistent with the pitch brightnesses of each. Again, we have considered yellow as joyous, violet as a melancholy color. The most joyous notes would accordingly be yellow-like and high, those of opposite quality blue-violet-like and low. The merriest sounds must be such high-pitched ones as those of children's or women's laughter; the saddest, those low-pitched ones found in moans, groans, etc. It will not be possible at very high pitch to produce an unambiguous effect of sadness, or an unambiguous effect of joy at a very low one. Is it not true that the higher notes of the soprano are either inexpressive or joyous, while the lower tones of the alto are either inexpressive or melancholy?

The whole question of sounds is difficult to investigate without very special apparatus. Furthermore, if it is true that only complex tones or timbres can be highly saturated or totally unsaturated, it follows that most loci on the sound solid will be represented by qualities which because of their blend character will exhibit a certain unclearness or ambiguity rendering their ascription to an exact locus on the solid more or less out of the question. But for the assumption of totally unique dimensions of auditory quality there seems no sufficient evidence. The same variables which account for color differences may, for all that we yet know, furnish the explanation of those of sound.

### SECTION 34. TOUCH, TEMPERATURE, AND PAIN

All skin sensations are somewhat difficult to observe. They lack the distinctness and the stability of visual qualities, and the attitude of observation is interfered with by marked tendencies toward behavior. We undergo pain as well as note its presence; pain in ourselves is ourselves in pain—that is to say, wholly detached contemplation of pain is not possible, any more than is such contemplation of an emotion. And tickle and itch exhibit this subjective and behavioristic character perhaps even more strongly. Extreme "psychic distance" is a priori impossible toward intrabodily experiences. Indeed, such distance would be identical with objectification in external space in the manner of colors or sounds.

It is the very essence of colors that they can be calmly, distinctly contemplated, and readily and accurately compared. It is the essence of most other sensations, even, to some extent, sounds, that they can be so treated only to a much lesser degree. One consequence is that with the non-visual sensations even the homogeneity of their quality through space is difficult to be sure of. Pain, for instance, may be a certain spatial pattern of qualities rather than a unitary quality like red or a given hue of orange. Warmth may be another such pattern, and the difference between warmth and pain may be a pattern difference rather than a difference of simple quality.

This hypothesis is borne out by the reports of Nafe's observers, who could find in cutaneous sensations only one simple quality, brightness, which they reported as common to all of these sensations.[17] Differences between heat, warmth, cold, pain, contact, itch, and tickle were described as differences in degree of, and spatio-temporal patterning of spots of, brightness. If this result is to be accepted, then all cutaneous sensations are gray, or graylike qualities, in varying configurations in space and time. The skin sense would be analogous to the most primitive mode of vision, that of the completely color-blind. There seems nothing unreasonable in this conception, which would certainly simplify the problem, and is in so far to be welcomed. But it is not quite clear whether the protocols justify the denial of chromatic variations to the cutaneous sensations. There may be such variations, but in such low degrees of saturation as to be readily overlooked, and yet of importance in contributing to the Gestalt aspects of the contrasts between warm and cold, or tickle and pain. When warmth is said to "glow," for instance, there is just possibly reference to a mildly saturated reddish or orangelike quality, which to me at least does seem often, if not always, to characterize this sensation. Cool seems more clearly unsaturated, paler as well as brighter. But again there may be a slight bluelike or greenish cast to the "bright spots" composing coolness.

Pain forms the most difficult problem. According to Pikler, tickle is greenlike, itch like yellow, and pain akin to red. It would follow that tickle should seem cooler than the others, particularly than pain. This seems to me the fact. But pain is re-

---

[17] J. P. Nafe, "Psychology of Felt Experience," *American Journal of Psychology*, XXXIX (1927), 367-89; "Dermal Sensitivity," *Pedagogical Seminary*, XXXIV (1927), 14-28.

ported as extremely bright, and in so far it cannot closely resemble red. However, there are pains and pains, and many deep, non-cutaneous ones at least may be definitely dull or dark. Perhaps the bright pains should be compared to pink? But here arises a baffling inconsistency. The unpleasantness which most bright pains display is in apparent contradiction to their brightness, for unpleasantness is unanimously reported in Nafe's protocols as dull or dark. Perhaps, after all, the unpleasantness of such pains is not intrinsic but concomitant. Perhaps the only reason why we usually dislike them is, as Nafe suggests, that certain motor responses of aversion are automatically set off by them. There are some pains whose intrinsic unpleasantness can, I believe, be distinctly intuited, but these are in my experience the dull, visceral pains. Bright pains, I confess, are a puzzle, from the standpoint of the affective theory of sensation.

### SECTION 35. TASTE AND SMELL

That tastes and smells are closely related in quality is a fact verified thrice a day by all of us. The taste and smell of an apple form a true blend as plainly as do the tastes of sweet and sour in lemonade, except that the former union is even more complete in that it is really much easier to distinguish the sweet-like and sourlike aspects of lemonade than the smell and taste constituents of an apple. In fact, it is easier to intuit a stronger likeness between these constituents, when once they have been distinguished, than between sweet and sour. An apple smells far more nearly as it tastes when smell is eliminated than as, say, quinine tastes. The smell and taste of vinegar are unmistakably alike. And there are equally clear instances of bitter-like smells, e.g., the skunk's odor. With the possible exception of salt, every taste has its smell correlate. With all the baffling difficulties which attempts to classify smells have thus far encountered, it is noteworthy that little use has been made of these analogies, although opportunity is thus given us of orienting the study of this difficult problem about the results secured in a much easier one.

It is, however, true that even this easier problem is far from completely solved. It is agreed that there are four taste primaries, as there are four primaries of chromatic color; that these are sweet, salt, sour, and bitter; and that, as in vision, intermediate qualities occur, by virtue of which all tastes form a continuum. But the boundaries of this continuum and the relative positions of tastes upon it are far from clearly made out, and of course the idea of treating the four critical tastes as polar opposites of two Cartesian variables has seldom been considered. According to the "gustatory tetrahedron" of Henning, indeed, polar opposition does not exist, and intermediaries between any two primary tastes are simply intermediate tastes, rather than, as in certain cases of vision, neutralized or non-saturated, as it were, gray tastes. Yet such non-saturated tastes have been detected, produced by mixing sweet and salt solutions.[18] It would appear that these tastes are complementary opposites. Here, then, is one of our co-ordinates. Nothing is left for the other but sour-bitter. The difficulty of verifying neutralization here may be due to the fact that gustatory localization is sufficiently vague to make it impossible to draw a sharp line introspectively between a sour-bitter occupying the same portion of phenomenal space and a pattern of adjacent sour and bitter spots. It will perhaps be conceded, however, that the most unmistakable saturated intermediates of taste are sweet-sour (lemonade), sweet-bitter (chocolate candy), salt-bitter (Epsom salts), salt-sour (salt pickles). "Sweet-salt" seems meaningless, and "sour-bitter" problematic. The second is suggested by grapefruit, but whether—as suggested above—by adjacent areas is the question. On the whole, the best working hypothesis is that proposed by Pikler,[19] according to which the following order obtains:

SWEET

BITTER   SOUR

SALT

[18] See F. Kiesow, "Zur physiologischen Psychologie des Geschmacksinnes," *Philosophische Studien*, XII, 255–78.

[19] *Op. cit.*, IV, 63.

This corresponds formally with the order of colors, with saturated intermediates, analogous to orange, etc., in sweet-sour, sour-salt, salt-bitter, bitter-sweet, while sweet-salt and sour-bitter correspond to the complementary pairs of primary colors. Pikler considers the analogy as material as well as formal, and regards salt as a sort of gustatory yellow (on the ground of its sharpness or brightness), sour as gustatory green, sweet as blue-like (because of its mildness and dulness), red as akin to bitter (both being duller than yellow or salt, but "rougher" than green or sour).[20] One objection to this is that bitter seems distinctly darker than sweet, whereas red is brighter than blue. On the other hand, I at least have always felt something sweetlike in blue, something mild and caressing. Starting from the color, I could arrive at no other taste as its analogue, and the same is no less true of the green affinity of sour. For red and yellow only bitter and salt would remain; the brightness of salt would suggest yellow while the darkness of bitter would absolutely exclude this color. Moreover, this darkness cannot be much in excess of that appropriate to the correlate of red, for the intensity of bitterness is too marked. Thus I do not see how to improve upon Pikler's doctrine even though I am dissatisfied with it. It assumes the usual color primaries instead of the scarlet, buttercup, sea-green, and violet which seem to me more accurate. Yet for these heterodox primaries I can see no plausible analogues among the taste primaries as generally conceived or as I am able to conceive them.

If the basic scheme which we have so far applied to saturated qualities, to qualities of chroma in a generalized sense, is applied to tastes, serious difficulties arise. That sour is cool in comparison to bitter seems observable enough, but that sweet is the opposite of joyous, and salt the maximum of this variable, is far indeed from clear to me.

Perhaps a comparison of tastes with odors will help us here. The best classification of odors is generally conceded to be that of Henning. Yet the unsatisfactoriness of his scheme is also widely acknowledged. The most searching critique of Henning's

[20] *Ibid.*, p. 50.

theory has been made by Pikler, who has proposed a radical simplification of it, the result of which is a thoroughgoing parallelism between taste and smell.[21] For sweet we have among odors fragrant or flowery; for sour, "vinegary"; for bitter, foul; for salt, burning. Of these odors only vinegary is lacking in Henning's list of six (plainly because he has no interest in taste analogies), but of the other five, fruity, spicy, and resinous are regarded as compounds or intermediates. Fruity is analyzed as fragrant and vinegary, or sweet and sour; spicy as sweet and burning, in some cases with a trace of sour or foul; resinous as sweet, sour, and burning. It is interesting that the taste and smell of fruit should, upon this hypothesis, turn out to be so closely related. Acid and sugar are of course the characteristic taste constituents of fruit. That fruity, spicy, and flowery all have an aspect of fragrance or sweetness in common seems evident enough. If the comparison of burning with salt can be accepted, the result is the most promising unification and simplification of the system of chemical sensations yet proposed. That Henning should have overlooked the possibility of reducing the olfactory primaries to four is not hard to explain. For he gives no sharp definition of the concept of primacy, such as would serve to bring the influence of associations—nowhere more powerful than with smells—under control. It is natural, for example, that fruity odors should be thought of as basic, for one does not easily think of fruits as unimportant among the kinds of substances. Concerning spices the same can be said.[22]

A cardinal defect in Henning's scheme is the neglect of the brightness axis. In all other senses besides the olfactory the partial dependence of qualitative upon intensive variations is so manifest that we should expect this to be true also of olfaction.

[21] *Ibid.*, pp. 38-49. Since writing the foregoing I have learned that practically the same scheme as Pikler's has been arrived at independently by two commercial chemists, who find it a quite satisfactory classification for chemical purposes (see E. C. Crocker and L. F. Henderson, "Analysis and Classification of Odors," *American Perfumer and Essential Oil Review*, August, 1927; for a sympathetic discussion of their view see Boring, *American Journal of Psychology*, XL, 345). See also Crocker and Henderson, "Whiff Numbers," *The Technology Review*, 1934, pp. 171-72.

[22] Strong evidence of the composite character of most common odors is given by Hoffman, *Zeitschrift für Biologie*, 1921, pp. 28-66.

In a remarkable recent paper impressive experimental evidence is presented for the view that odors can be classified according to an attribute closely resembling the pitch of tones, and also, though to a lesser degree, the brightness of colors. "Odor-pitch" is proposed as the fundamental variable of olfaction.[23]

If Pikler's scheme is correct, then sweet-burnt and acid-foul odors should produce neutralization, subject to the localization difficulty referred to in discussing complementary tastes. "Flat" or neutral odors do seem to occur, as anyone can find by entering a laundry.

The active-passive or warm-cold axis fits, at least roughly, the contrast of bitter and sour, foul and acid, red and green (although, once more, bitter seems dark, like brown rather than red). But the sweet-salt, fragrant-burnt dimension, which Pikler connects with the contrast of blue-yellow, seems to me about as convincing or unconvincing if read the other way—i.e., to correspond to yellow-blue, which I have construed as joy-sorrow. The difficulty with this latter reading is that salt is apparently too bright, which is one of Pikler's reasons for reversing the analogy. Probably the truth is somewhat intricate; which does not necessarily mean that we must fall back after all into the conventional view of total uniqueness of quality in each sensory mode. Such blind unintelligibility is always open to us as a desperate last resort, but there is nothing desperate in the failure of a few inquirers to carry out a radically untraditional program of research with more than very limited success. The discovery of a possible simplification of odor classifications and of two unmistakably clear similarities between odor and taste is success enough to encourage us to continue in the endeavor. Let anyone smell acetic acid or certain sweet-smelling chemicals and see if he can see more than the very slightest qualitative difference between these odors and sour or sweet tastes. He will even note, I predict, that "sweet" is a more appropriate word than "fragrant" for certain smells, fragrance suggesting addi-

---

[23] A. Juhasz, A szagerzetek egy uj tuloj densaga, *Athenaeum*, XII (1926), 34–39 (I am indebted to Mr. Stephen Chak Tornay for an oral translation of this important article); and, in German, Juhasz, *Neunter Kongress für experimentelle Psychologie* (1925), and the Eighth International Congress of Psychology.

tional features found indeed in the odor of flowers but not in the chemicals in question.

## SECTION 36. THE GENERAL QUESTION

The aim of this and of the preceding sections in this chapter has been to suggest how sensory qualities from widely different modes may be seen as values of variables common to all modes, and to all experience actual or possible. These variables we have conceived as those of intensity, activity-passivity, joy-sorrow, duration, and spatial extension; and we have sought to deduce these from the concept of social feeling, feeling of feeling, as such. In attempting to identify these variables in the various sensory fields we have met with difficulties whose resolution only the future can provide. The possible sources of these difficulties are various. The number of variables required may be greater; indeed, the question is worth asking whether, considering "all possible qualities," the dimensions should not be conceived as infinite. This infinity would not conflict with the assumption that all qualities fall upon one ultimate continuum of potentiality, but it would render the application of this idea to the facts of our experience a difficult and perhaps almost useless procedure. It is, however, never science to accept a larger number of variables than we are forced to do by the facts. We know from colors that sense qualities involve not less than five dimensions: space, time, strength or brightness, a factor separating red from green, and a similar factor separating yellow from blue. We ought to hope that these very factors will suffice to account for the qualities intuited by means of the other senses. That this hope is about to be realized would be an extravagant conclusion from the considerations set forth in this chapter. But it does, I think, follow from these considerations that the possession by any of the senses of a mode of variation additional to the five mentioned has not as yet been proved or disproved; and that the question involves subtleties quite beyond the reach of traditional approaches to the problem. The discoveries by Nafe of the rôle of spatio-temporal pattern alone in differentiating sensations of the skin show how utterly naïve it is to rely upon our offhand impressions of qualitative uniqueness as decisive for the number of variables which sensory experience embodies. For spatio-temporal pattern is common to all the sensory realms.

There seems but one justifiable verdict—the question calls for further study, particularly, perhaps, experimental study. It may be also that we need to form clearer conceptions than anyone now has concerning the logical aspects of qualitative continuity and discontinuity, concerning the nature of qualitative comparison.

# CHAPTER VIII
# SENSATION AND ENVIRONMENT
\*\*

*My objection to pluralistic systems which hold that the distinction between different minds, or between mind and matter, is irreducible . . . . is just that they proclaim problems to be insoluble merely because three thousand years of thought by a few members of a species which may have many hundred million years ahead of it has not yet solved them. . . . . Monism has the advantage that if it is wrong it will ultimately lead to self-contradiction, whereas dualistic systems, which purport to give a less complete account of the world, are therefore less susceptible of disproof. . . . . We can only discern a little mind in a dog, and at present none in an oyster or an oak. Nevertheless . . . . if we ever explain life and mind in terms of atoms, I think we shall have to attribute to the atoms the same nature as that of minds or constituents of mind such as sensations.*

J. B. S. HALDANE

*Consciousness is a sort of public spirit among the nerve cells.*

CHARLES S. PEIRCE

\*\*

### SECTION 37. THE PSYCHO-PHYSICAL PROBLEM

THERE is at least one dimension of sensory quality whose correlation with its physiological conditions need not be regarded as essentially mysterious, a mere "parallelism" or inexplicable conjunction. This is intensity or "brightness." For, intensity being physiologically identified as time density of the all-or-none impulses of nerve activity, what could be more intelligible than that the consciousness of time density should be intensity? If the frequencies are too high to be separately distinguished, they will naturally fuse in consciousness into a smooth stream whose energy per unit of time is proportional to the number of pulses. And yet, it will be said, what can there be in common between physical and psychic energy? And then there are the other qualitative variables. Surely they at least have no physical analogues!

The only answer I am able to suggest falls under the general head of "panpsychism." If nerve cells are living and sentient, then the "warmth," "pleasantness," etc., of human sensation may not be without its parallel in the sentience of these cells. Facts bearing upon this hypothesis are neither totally lacking nor, as yet, even remotely adequate to its verification. Here I merely point out that affective characters express volitional tendencies, that these are embodied in behavior, that cells in some measure and fashion behave, that therefore the hypothesis that when the man suffers his cells also endure negative feeling is in principle open to observational test. This is enough to render the hypothesis a legitimate speculation, and to refute the contention that panpsychism has no implications for research.[1] The observation of cell behavior can hardly prove a waste of time; panpsychism gives us a clue to this behavior which, vague though it be, cannot if applied critically do much harm, and which no one can know will not sooner or later prove fruitful in physiological inquiry. Let us then take seriously the view that a cell is not only a living but a sentient organism. It has no nervous system, you may object, therefore it has no consciousness and no sentience. It has no stomach, I reply, therefore it cannot digest food; no lungs, therefore it cannot absorb oxygen; no afferent and motor nerves, therefore it cannot respond and adapt itself to its environment; no reproductive organs, therefore it cannot multiply its kind, etc. If these inferences are not valid, and they cannot be, since their premisses are true and their conclusions false to the facts, then neither is the former reasoning supporting the dependence of sentience upon a nervous system coercive.[2] Lack of explicit organ does not spell lack of function, but primitive form of the function. If anyone could show that sentience as such involves more complexity than a microbe possesses structurally, we should have to admit that

[1] See Morris R. Cohen, *Reason and Nature* (New York, 1931), p. 307.

[2] The most cogent statement known to me of a contrary view is given by Marston, King, and Marston, *Integrative Psychology*, p. 6. But this statement is only seemingly in conflict with panpsychism. The possibility that, apart from animals with nerves, the sentient unit may be the single cell is not discussed.

the microbe cannot feel. But I do not see that the idea of feeling posits any greater complexity than even an electron exhibits.

The cell, therefore—so our account begins—is a creature that feels. Moreover, it does not feel just itself, its own life. For its life is its feeling, and then there must be something for it to feel, not just its feeling. Moreover, since cells are grouped in highly specialized interacting communities, we infer that the feeling which is their essence and motive force must be largely under the tyrannical dominance of "mob psychology," group feeling running in rather fixed or habitual grooves. The cells act together because they feel together, because waves of almost identical feeling pervade and hold them in *rapport* with one another. The ground of this *rapport* is the same in principle as that which holds nature generally together. Some will leap at once to the idea of a divine feeling, the ultimate focus and control of the total sympathetic connectedness. But in the case of multicellular animals an intermediate principle is involved. The animal as a whole is individually sentient. Its feeling, likewise social, is peculiarly sensitive to, participant in, the feelings of its nerve cells. A wave of mob feeling in these appears in it as a single similarly toned feeling. Thus with prevailingly pained cells in some portion of the nervous system, the animal feels pain, more or less localized as the wave of painful feeling involves a larger or smaller area in the total cellular community. The problem of interaction, of a physical change producing a mental, and vice versa, becomes, for the first time, something more than a blind mystery. The cells have their own individuality and minute independence or spontaneity of feeling. They depend, moreover, in part upon sentient units composing the external environment; for with these likewise, to a greater or less but never to a zero degree, they are in *rapport*. A wave of feeling outside the body is sympathetically prolonged within it —modified, however, by some degree of reaction—and becomes as thus modified further prolonged and further modified in the same manner into a feeling of the total animal itself. The reverse process is on the same principles. The difference is that the animal as a whole has a larger degree of freedom; for it has the power to act sympathetically to an effective extent upon a vast multitude of organisms simultaneously, to play like an organist upon the whole complexus of feeling units composing the body, whereas the effective control of any single cell is only upon its immediate neighbors. To depend upon the body is thus to be constituted by sympathy with it, particularly certain parts of it which themselves participate responsively in the remaining parts and, both directly and indirectly, with the external world.

An advantage of this view is that it enables us to answer the otherwise embarrassing question: If a sensation is a mode of immediate intuition, of what is it immediately aware? The answer—of redness, or whatever the sensory quality may be—is hardly sufficient. A quality qualifies something. What, we must ask, is immediately given as red? If it be said, "Simply the sensory experience itself," then we have an absolute solipsism with respect to immediacy, and all accounts of our knowledge of a real world are doomed from the start. But if it be said rather, "It is the red book which is immediately intuited as red," then we have to explain away utterly one of the most certain of scientific facts, the primary dependence of the red sensation upon something quite other than the book, namely, the nervous process. Surely the hypothesis which most simply resumes our knowledge here is that the immediate object of sensory intuitions is that upon which they most directly depend. If anything is directly known to be qualified by redness, it is one's own body when seeing red. We have to take account of the dependence and the givenness; it is scientifically inadmissible to assume that these are anything more than two ways of viewing one and the same relation until this, the simplest, conception of the situation has been given a thorough trial. Modern thought has by no means accorded it this trial, but has favored instead almost every conceivable alternative. If dependence is givenness, and immediate dependence is immediate givenness, then what we intuit as red is the state of our own nerves together with the state of the environment in so far as the latter is inseparably contained in the former by virtue of the organic unity of the physical world. This doubtless includes the book, but only to a minor degree, since a very similar nervous process would be possible with a very different physical object or with no definite external stimulation at all. Primarily it is the bodily cells, then the light-rays, then finally the book, which are red.

The obvious objection to this view is that it is the book, and not the nerves, which seems red, and that the immediately given is what seems or appears and as it appears. One may further observe that the nerves do not seem to be immediately given at all, but are known only by highly indirect inference. The assumption from which this criticism derives its pertinence is that immediate and clear intuitions are by definition the same. If the nerves are given, it is with such unclearness that for detailed knowledge of them we are almost entirely dependent upon inference. When inference has built up a detailed picture of the nervous process, it is not strange that we should fail to recognize that these are the very things we have directly experienced all our lives. Yet there are certain details, unfortunately as yet but meagerly supplied, by which the identity of the subjects of the picture and of the experience might be perceived. But the important point is that a sensory experience is no mere registration of an object, in the body or out of it, but an incipient adaptation and reaction to the immediately felt fact—a reaction molded by the past fortunes of the individual and species and its life-goals. We feel chiefly, though not solely (since nature is one), what goes on in brain and eye, but we *mean* what is transpiring quite elsewhere. If it were otherwise, we could be subject to no illusions, but we should also possess no knowledge. We should feel what we felt, and all else would be nothing to us. Not that meaning projects outward what is merely inward, for nothing is merely anywhere ("fallacy of simple location"), but that meaning enormously enlarges upon the clearness with which the outward is present in the body and in immediate intuition. It does so at its own peril, and as taught by experience and adaptation.

There are many philosophers who concede all this. But not all of them take pains to render the facts intelligible. If it is primarily the nerves which are red, how is this to be conceived? In what sense do the red-seeing optic nerve and brain become red? We can declare this an ultimate mystery, or we can hold that it is self-explanatory. To me at least neither contention has anything to do with the attitude which promotes scientific understanding, except as a purely temporary device to concentrate attention on more pressing matters. What is a nerve like when it is qualified by red? The affective theory of sensation, coupled with the hypothesis that the nerves are individually sentient, provides a straightforward answer. Red is a mode of feeling value, describable in terms of the dimensions of social affectivity as such. The nerve cells have feelings also determinable on these dimensions. The relation between red as we see it and red as it is in the nerves is the relation between the individual units of a complex of feelings and the complex as a single over-all quality. The characters of units and complex will not be the same, but they may none the less possess very real similarity. For instance, the mere fact that a thousand units of cellular suffering were so blurred together into a single fusion or timbre that the individual units lost their distinctness from the standpoint of the fusion would give no ground for the alteration of the feeling quality from that of suffering to that of pleasure. Many pleasures blurred together could only, it seems, produce a single blurred pleasure. Thus, with all the vast differences, inference from our human subjective state to that of its immediately though vaguely given objects, the somatic cells, is possible.[3]

As for the book, it is probably, in no comparably pregnant sense, red at all. For it is very clear that what goes on in the bodily cells is primarily determined by the past history and innerbodily environment of these cells, and only in second instance by the impinging mechanical and radiant stimulation, more indirectly still by the objects from which these stimuli may come. That the cells feel individually what we vaguely feel as a blurred synthesis, is, on our theory, inevitable, for this is sim-

[3] This is Whitehead's doctrine of "transmutation" (see *Process and Reality*, pp. 384 ff.).

ply the mind-body relation; but that the molecules of the red book should be feeling as the cells of the optic-nerve circuit feel is a very different matter indeed.

There is, however, an old argument upon this point. If the book is not in any pregnant sense red, then our senses are systematic deceivers to a degree that we dislike to admit. But this argument simply raises the question: What, after all, are the senses trying to tell us; what sort of information is it their function to impart? Is the eye really saying to us, "This book, as a physical object in its trans-human existence, *is* red"? Or is the eye perhaps saying, "This book, as an entity of service to human beings for certain purposes, is red"? Which view is the more in accord with our biological knowledge?

It is true, no doubt, that no perception of the book could be of service unless it did impart information about the book as it really is. But it is an old insight, upon which all modern control of nature is based, that the only detailed information of this sort is given not directly by the secondary qualities, such as red, but by what, for this very reason, are known as the primary qualities. The book really is larger than a fly, and it really is longer than it is wide, in a sense in which it is not really any particular color. The redness of the book may then have three kinds of significance. It reveals, in considerable detail, the shape, and, more indirectly perhaps, other primary qualities. Then it may reveal, also in somewhat particular terms, the utility of the book for basic (primitive) human purposes. To this topic we return in the next section. And, finally, the redness may reveal, though in highly general terms only, the quality, not indeed of the book in particular, but of physical objects as such. This third possibility means that books and other things like them may actually have secondary as well as primary qualities— and have them not by virtue of the presence of human percipients—but that these qualities need not be the particular ones we sense them as having. The real quality of the book may be very different indeed from red, and, for all our perception of it as red proves, may have a quality actually somewhat more like green. Assuming the affective theory of sensation, the possession by physical things of qualities which in general, though not necessarily in particular, are like those we perceive amounts, of course, to the doctrine of panpsychism.[4]

The above-mentioned three kinds of conceivable significance attaching to the sensory qualities are those which could be supposed invariably to obtain. There is a fourth kind which may obtain in certain cases but not in others. If an automobile brake emits a shriek or groan, we do not suppose that the brake is in agony. One may suppose, indeed, that our own auditory nerve cells are suffering, but this is another matter. If, however, a human being or animal utters the shriek, we may very well suppose suffering like that qualifying the sound to inhere in the source of the sound.

Here are four ways in which the sense qualities may be true characterizations of the environment. Is that not enough to exonerate the senses from the charge of systematic deception? If, however, we abandon the affective account of these qualities, we shall either grant this charge or posit a completely unintelligible inherence of an ineffable redness or loudness in the physical world, either by itself or as containing the human percipient. How the addition of the latter brings about the existence of the quality we shall regard as beyond explanation.

In view of the purposive character of the sensory response it is to be presumed that the most important function of a sensory quality, besides the all-important one of outlining the primary qualities, must be that of indicating in a qualitative way its value for human life. Sugar really is sweet, in the sense that this positive affective quality expresses the objective fact of the nutritious nature of this substance. This is the clue which we have to examine in detail in the next section.

SECTION 38. SENSE QUALITIES AND ADAPTATION

That immediately intuited qualities may serve to adapt the organism to its environment is evidenced by pleasure and pain, which seem of themselves to induce opposite behavioristic modes of acceptance and rejection, under circumstances which

[4] See sec. 39.

in the main render these activities appropriate. But few seem to have ascribed this third mode of adaptiveness to the simple qualities of external sensation. Any quality whatever, it seems to be held, could have conveyed the behavioristic meaning of red—such as danger signal, rose, anger, embarrassment, etc.—, just as well as red, if only it had occurred constantly in the same contexts as those in which red has actually been found. To be sure, some thinkers have held with crude common sense that only red could have been appropriate, inasmuch as the physical objects in question are themselves red, possess the same quality as the sensation. But the biological significance of this view is hard to see, since it is not the color of an object, in this sense of a simple quality, which is relevant to the fate of the organism, but rather certain underlying physical forces and complexes whose nature seems by no resemblance or logical relationship to be indicated by the quality.

The question stands at once in a new light if the doctrine of sensory affectivity is taken seriously. If redness is essentially an objectified feeling attitude, akin to pleasure or pain, then the question of its behavioristic appropriateness becomes the question of whether or not the emotional content of red corresponds to the average practical significance of the principal objects of nature which reflect the longer rays of the spectrum. That the qualities of one sense possess this appropriateness has been remarked by one psychologist at least.[5] The most positive emotionality in the sphere of taste is sweetness; and there is no class of objects in nature that are so uniformly nutritious and wholesome as those that taste sweet. The most negative gustatory quality is bitterness; and the bitter substances include many poisonous and non-nutritious plants. Sour and salt are intermediate both affectively[6] and nutritively, their relative order being perhaps a little ambiguous. The question which obviously suggests itself is whether similar principles apply to all the senses.

[5] I refer to my former teacher, L. T. Troland, whose remarks in a class lecture first suggested to me the view which follows.
[6] See Beebe-Center, *Pleasantness and Unpleasantness*, pp. 144 ff.

The facts which reveal the adaptive value of the sensory qualities are, for the most part, well known. But they have been interpreted in such fashion as entirely to obscure this implication. I refer to all those facts which have been held to confirm an associational explanation of the aesthetic content of sense qualities. Thus, if green is cool, this is said to be simply because green foliage has been experienced in connection with protection from the sun's heat. Now that the facts do suggest a connection, which might perhaps be called an "association," based upon past experience, as the basis of the emotional qualities of colors and other sense data, I am inclined to believe. But I do not believe that the most illuminating interpretation of this connection is one which posits a duality of emotional and sensory quality, but rather one which asserts their identity.

The ordinary associational doctrine conceives as terms of the connection in question two entities, both of which are directly given and psychological. The association, in short, is between "ideas." The doctrine I wish to suggest is that the most fundamental associations are not in this fashion intra-psychological but psycho-physical. One and only one term of the relation is a state of the human psyche; and the other is a state of the physical environment, namely, the stimulus. Now sensation is beyond doubt a means whereby two factors are brought into connection on the basis of past (racial) experience, the external or environmental situation, and the internal psychological response. If, then, the response is, say, a feeling characterizable as cool—the sensation green, for example—then the mechanism which habitually sets off this response under certain external conditions may be said to associate the feeling of coolness, not with the sense datum green—for that is the coolness itself—but with light-rays of a certain wave-length. Assuming the affective theory of sensation, the only inborn factor that need be supposed in the sensing of the trees as green and cool in color is simply the sensory mechanism itself. The fact to be explained is not, upon this assumption, why red, in the psychological sense, is warm, for that is like asking why a circle is round. The question is rather why red in the physical sense—that is, light-radiations of a certain frequency—should occasion the sense datum red and not the sense datum green or blue, and this again is identical with the question as to why such radiations should be responded to visually with that objectified warm feeling we call "red" rather than with the opposite feeling we call "green."

The usual view of the emotional aspects of sensations as accretions added to them after they were otherwise fully constituted is a profoundly unbiological doctrine. For the basis of these emotionalities is fully as old in the world as the sense organs themselves. The experience of the beneficent effects of moderate light, for example, is incomparably older than vision itself. Surely we should expect such things to explain not simply how certain responses could be added to the sensations of color once on the scene, but also the very evolution and nature of these sensations, what they biologically and psychologically are.

#### A. VISION AND BEHAVIOR

The distribution of colors in the natural environment exhibits a plan so strikingly simple and clear in its broad outlines that glimpses of this plan were long ago perceived by philosophers. The plan is as follows. Barring biologically insignificant details, green is in nature the color of vegetable life and hence of the normal foreground; blue is the color of distant masses (the horizon, mountains, sky, and large bodies of water), hence of the normal background (including, to some extent, shadows); red is the color of blood, representing food, danger, death, combat; yellow is the color of sunlight; white, with yellow, the color of light, but further of snow and so of the winter landscape; black is the color of deep shadows and lowering clouds, the color of night and the absence of light, the color of ignorance, uncertainty, difficulty, danger, mystery, storm, and the absence of the life-giving solar energy, in which all higher animals delight to bathe themselves.

The connection of yellow with sunlight can be seen by observing the yellowish tinge of foliage or grass in a sunlit clearing as compared with that in the shaded forest. Thus we may say that blue-green is the color of the normal moderately lighted foreground, and yellow-green of the foreground in brilliant sunlight. For surely a foreground whose color is not primarily determined by vegetation and light is the exception, even in non-tropical countries, if we except the arctic regions, which are not the probable original home of man. In bright sunlight there is also a tendency toward white, but the only systematic occurrence of pure white is found in snow, and in the lighter clouds. The latter are of little practical account; but the snow-covered landscape is the outstanding color index of cold, and cold is a fundamental factor. Blackness is found in certain rocks and soils, certain tree trunks, and the hair of some animals and races of man; but all this is haphazard and incidental compared to the universal tendency of shadows (including that shadow of the earth itself, night) toward this color, which psychologists have been so eager to describe, with unconscious half-truth, as "no less positive" than the remaining colors.

Such is the classification of colors according to the biologically important objects which reflect them. We have now to analyze the specific character of this biological importance in each case, in order that we may compare it with the emotional significance of the respective colors.

The vegetable covering of the normal foreground is not for the most part, to man or to animals akin to man, of direct significance as food or danger or other vital condition. It affords shade and at the same time reflects the sun's rays with less loss of brightness than do distant objects. It is in no way an exciting fact, but a harmless and agreeable one. Those plants that are important as food, and those dangerous as poisons, are in neither case especially represented as a class by the color green. In short, the green vegetable covering of the earth is just the normal fact of existence. Psychologically, then, we should expect green to appear as a feeling of quiet cheerfulness. Who does not feel this to be in fact the character of green?

The behavioristic significance of the blue background is partly that of mere background and partly that of sky—that is to say, the source of light and the limit of the upward dimension of space, the realm of illumination and of triumph over gravity.

However, these two blues are not the same, since the violet and the purple of distant hills is very different from the far brighter blue of the usual clear sky. The blue of seas and lakes is the reflection of that of the sky and is of far less independent significance. Bodies of water can be recognized as such for all primordial needs apart from this color, which indeed does not attach to them except on clear days. On the other hand, the blue sky as an index of clear weather might impress itself even upon animals. The experience of that blue is bound up inseparably with that of an abundance of light, and is itself a luminous, "ethereal" blue. Nevertheless, neither the sky nor the distant land is an object of important and frequent direct reaction. The one thing to do about them, normally speaking, is to pay them no attention. A strong preoccupation with them as objects of vision might easily and frequently have fatal results with no likelihood of as frequent compensating advantages. On the psychological side this implies a desiderated lack of insistency or aggressiveness in blue as a datum of sense. Blue should not seem too clamorous or lively; it should "take a back seat" throughout. This it does by virtue of its blend of passivity (green) and somberness (violet).

Red offers perhaps the simplest problem of all. No other color can compare with it in the systematic way in which it stands for the dramatic crises of life, among all the higher animals. It is not merely that arterial blood, the central life-fluid, is of that color. We have to remember also that from the standpoint of vision it is chiefly by its color that blood is identified. Otherwise it cannot by sight be distinguished from water or other common fluids. Outside of vegetation nothing in nature probably is so readily and safely to be identified by its mere color as is the blood of the higher animals. But the identification of blood is the knowledge that edible flesh is at hand, or that foes or friends or members of the pack or the animal itself are in danger and pain. Blood is interwoven with success in the hunt, with consuming of the prey, with combat, and with being one's self, in person or in the group, preyed upon. Here are nearly all the great instinctive emotions, social solidarity, everything save sex, which depends visually upon form rather than color, and otherwise chiefly upon hearing and smell. What is life for a higher animal but a shedding of blood and a struggle to conserve his own or that of certain of his neighbors? If the color of blood is not to excite and move the higher animal, the remaining colors ought to put him to sleep! What, psychologically, do we find? That red is precisely the most dramatic and stirring of colors; that it lacks the light-hearted gaiety of yellow, the sunshine color; the cold intensity of white, the snow-and-cloud color; the quiet cheerfulness of green; the gentle affectionate quality of blue; and possesses, as no other color, the quality of excitement or activity. There is no other color which it is so necessary to take seriously.

There are two principal difficulties in the foregoing explanation of color. On the one hand, we have to conceive a mechanism whereby the adjustment of sensory response to environment can have come about. Here the inheritance of acquired characters and the survival of the fittest variations seem almost the only available principles, and of these the latter alone has much in biological knowledge to support it. The trouble is that it is hard to form even the vaguest estimate of the survival value involved in sensory affectivities, such as the coolness of green. We can only point, for instance, to the not infrequent instances in which constant contact with red has produced nervous exhaustion; and urge that the more primitive the man or the animal the more we should expect the influence of sensation to predominate over more sophisticated responses, such as the cognitive perception of the red object in terms of its causal implications. On the other hand, the entire reasoning proceeds upon the assumption that other modes of sensory response to the same stimuli would have been psycho-physically possible, even if biologically less useful or appropriate. But there must be a priori limits to what is possible, i.e., consistently conceivable. For instance, it cannot be wholly because of utility that light gives us the sense of intense activity, and darkness that of inactivity, which they do in fact arouse. For darkness is inactivity and light, intense activity, and the effect upon the organism is in mere logic bound to exhibit these facts. But here again we have no accurate measure of the extent of the possible as compared to the impossible situations. If and when we have so clarified our concepts that we see somewhat definitely into the a priori possibilities and into their relative utilities, we shall be in a position to reason with more confidence concerning the selective action of the struggle for survival upon the evolution of the senses.

### B. HEARING

The biological function of sound is, at least in degree if not in kind, unique. The clue to this uniqueness is seen if we consider the situation of an animal totally deaf. There seems to be only one important difference which this handicap would make to the animal. Adjustment to the inorganic and vegetable world would go on much as usual. To be sure, wind, waves, and landslides could no longer be identified by their audible effects, but touch and vision would as a rule supply all necessary information in regard to these things. But consider the animal's relations to the rest of the animal world. How seriously would these be impeded! It could be taken by surprise by an animal approaching from the lee side, it could not be called to its mate or young, it could not adequately convey a combat-saving warning to any foe or sex rival who should underestimate its pugnacity. In short, its control over its relations to its animal fellows would be seriously impoverished. We may express the uniquely social character of hearing by remarking that it is the only sense organ whose important responses are almost entirely brought forth by stimuli produced by other animals. This means, from an evolutionary standpoint, that the adaptation of responsive organism to stimulus may here be met more or less halfway by an adaptation of stimulus to response. Evolution here has its grip not only upon the reception of the stimulus but also upon its production. This double control is also found in other senses—in vision and smell particularly. In so far, for example, as coloration is sex lure or camouflage or symbol of herd unity, it is of this social type. But on the whole it is not mainly by color that social relationships are realized, except in the case of blood-red, and here the chemical needs of the organism determine, I take it, the structure of the hemoglobin so that here the social reference could hardly have played any part in the evolution of the stimulating factor. In the main, coloration is social chiefly as camouflage—that is, its purpose is really antisocial, not to reveal environing animal life, but to conceal it. Smells are either inevitable by-products of the necessary chemistry of the body or else are sex lures or warning signals against attack or deterrents to consumption as food (skunk, stinkbugs). But these latter, the social instances, cannot well determine the systematic meanings of odors, since the primary function of smell must be to detect the presence of the chemically more or less inevitable bodily odors, and so to identify friend, foe, or quarry, and, further, to report upon the edibility of foods. In hearing alone, where the stimuli are produced largely by the contraction of muscles whose action is capable of endless variability without essentially altering the basic chemical and organic plan of the species, do we find life in a position largely to control the major stimuli with reference to their social effect. And yet, even here, we must not pass lightly over the question as to how free from organic necessities these variations are. Could a cat in a state of peaceful pleasure, as when being stroked, growl fiercely, as it does when disturbed while gnawing a bone? How could a general placidity be made physiologically consistent with the tense state of lung muscles and vocal cords necessarily involved in growling? We see clearly that the evolution of emotional expression does not, as it were, have its hands entirely free to alter the stimulus side of the communication, any more than we can see how an ear could readily evolve which would hear physically intense sounds as faint, and vice versa. From the standpoint of bodily engineering, there are limits, at least of convenience, set to these things. However, if we concede that neither vocal cords nor ear were physiological necessities, apart from the need to communicate, the need for language and social awareness, we will not hesitate to grant also that the exact form and functioning of both receiving and sending organs must also be partly contingent upon, hence possibly rendered adaptive to, these functions.

It is a remarkable fact that the cries of the higher animals are intelligible, in their demonstrable behavioristic meanings, apart from the necessity for learning these meanings from further experience of such animals. No musician could fail to discriminate between the discontented "meow" of the cat and the sense of delicious pleasure in those soft purling sounds, quite distinct from purring, which experience adequately yet superfluously shows to denote pleasure or contentment. I say superfluously, for the hearing of the sound conveys the meaning at once and directly. We should be astonished, upon first hearing it, if the creature should at the same time behave in a manner inconsistent with this interpretation, which we could not avoid making if we really attended to the sound.

The cries of distress of dog or cat, of bird or human being, all show a family likeness. When the nest is being robbed, the parent-birds do not sing or merely utter usual call notes. Their voices take on strained, distressful, plaintive tones appropriate, to any human ears, to the situation. The songs, on the other hand, are usually joyous. But there are exceptions—that of the wood pewee, for instance, which is strangely minor and plaintive. Still even these are not really distressful. Now birds do not sing when there is reason to think them physiologically depressed, but only in a mood of exaltation—frequently, to be sure, that of the "joy of battle"—as evidenced by behavior.

#### C. THERMAL SENSATIONS

Suppose that in the presence of what from the physical standpoint is called "cold" the animal responded with the sensation which psychologically is called "warmth," and that in the presence of mild physical warmth the animal felt cold. Now although both warm and cold as sensations shade into pain, there is an intrinsic likeness, noted by Nafe's subjects,[7] between warm and pleasantness, and between cold and unpleasantness. Hence the hypothetical reversal of these responses implies a reversal of these affectivities such that the animal would be en-

[7] See "An Experimental Study of the Affective Qualities," *American Journal of Psychology*, 1924, p. 520.

couraged to prolong the exposure to cold and shorten that to warmth. This, from the adaptive standpoint, would be the reversal of the appropriate behavior. It follows that the actual correlation of stimulus and response is in a broad way in accordance with adaptive requirements. The exposure to warmth which falls short of heat is incomparably more advantageous than that to cold of a degree to be felt (through the fur or other protective covering) as cold. The feeling tones of the two sensations are the faithful conscious expression of these facts.

It is sometimes stated that all sensory qualities, when very intense, become painful in character. This statement is highly inaccurate, to say the least. Bright light may hurt the eyes and so cause pain, but the pain is clearly distinct and by several careful observers has been sharply distinguished from the brightness sensation itself.[8] Again, sweet taste in itself never hurts; even though saccharine, by producing an after-taste of bitter, may be disagreeable. Or, still again, very high sounds hurt the ears, but the pain sensation here is tactual, not auditory. But hot and cold become more and more like pain as their intensity increases, until finally they have literally become sheer pain. Nothing could be more fitting in the biological sense. For extreme heat and cold are highly dangerous factors in the environment, and few things could be more necessary than that they should be repulsive to the organism. The danger, moreover, like the painfulness, is a matter of degree.

It is not, however, necessary to suppose that the sensations are what they are because of their fitness. Another explanation is possible. The temperature at which heat is felt as pain—like the pressure at which contact is so felt—is one at which the tissue, including perhaps the nervous tissue itself, begins to be damaged.[9] Now damage to a nerve cell, on our hypothesis, means pain or distress felt by the nerve cell as a sentient individual, and our human sensation as conditioned by the cell will be a sympathetic echo of its distress in fusion with echoes from a number of other cells. Hence if we are to sense

---

[8] See, e.g., Brentano, *Psychologie vom empirischen Standpunkt* (Leipzig, 1924), I, 214.
[9] Troland, *Sensation*, par. 407.

destructive temperatures or pressures at all, we must sense them as distressful or repugnant.

#### D. THE CHEMICAL SENSES AND PLEASURE AND PAIN

One of the most intensely positive of the objective feelings called sensations is the sweet odor of flowers. Yet what objects could be of less value to the organism than flowers? It would seem that only bees should have been equipped with this sensory response to them. We must note, however, that it is not flowers alone which are fragrant. The affinity of fruity odors to the flowery is stressed by Henning, and Pikler brilliantly explains fruity as simply a fragrant-sour (or flowery-vinegar) smell. Now it may be — the chemical facts are but partially known—that the odoriferous particles emitted by fruits and flowers are too much alike for a highly differential olfactory response to them to have been convenient. It would be interesting to compare the response of fruit-loving animals, such as bears, monkeys, and birds, to the odor of flowers with that of more purely carnivorous or grass-eating animals.[10]

Foul odors proceed from substances more or less injurious to man and to most animals. Carrion-eaters must, if the affective theory is true, have eccentric olfactory systems.

Vinegary odors come from acid substances harmful in large quantities or in concentrated form, but wholesome in dilute form, as in fruits. The negative affective tone is appropriately mild. It is worthy of note that the sweet-sour smell into which Pikler analyzes the fruity odor corresponds to the acid-sugar composition of fruits and to their taste. The acid taste and smell moderate the greed which a purely sweet one would release and thus lead to overconsumption of acid.

Of both taste and smell it is true that the very same factors which determine the value to the organism of the substances emitting the stimuli to these sensations may also be responsible for the immediate effect of benefit or injury to the receptor cells which I assume to be the basis of the affective content of the sensations. For both this immediate effect on the sense organs

---

[10] Some relevant data are given by Henning in *Der Geruch*, p. 262.

and the eventual effect of the substances when consumed as food are chemical, and in so far of the same order. Thus most poisons may damage the receiving apparatus of taste or smell or both before reaching and attacking more vital parts; and the sugary tastes or sweet odors may promote the local prosperity in the sensory region before their emitting substances have passed on to confer more fundamental benefits. When one considers how relatively unspecific most poisons are in respect to the various forms of protoplasm, and how equally universal is the value of many nourishing materials, such as sugars, one can perhaps concede some weight to such a hypothesis.

From the same standpoint we may consider the much-mooted question of the biological significance of pleasure and pain. There has been much controversy concerning whether or not pain always denotes a harmful and pleasure a helpful situation. The majority opinion seems to be that these generalizations must be qualified by numerous exceptions. But a minority argues that the exceptions need be admitted only if by harmful or helpful we mean to the organism as a whole and in the long run, whereas no exceptions need be made to the statement that pain means at least a local injury or hindrance, and pleasure at least a local success or facilitation. Even though a substance (such as sugar of lead) be eventually poisonous, it may temporarily favor the functioning of the gustatory apparatus and so taste sweet. Representatives of the majority view regard this claim as too unverified, or even too lacking in determinable meaning (how does sweet facilitate taste any more than salt or bitter?), to deserve serious consideration. Yet this defect is not necessarily incurable. It might be possible to detect a favorable action of sugar of lead upon sensory cells, and there is already some evidence supporting the view that pain denotes incipient destruction of nerve cells. The fact that pain acts like a fatigue reaction, occurring after a slight delay or violent stimulation, is clearly such evidence. Moreover, pain-related sensations, such as bitter or hot or cold, are already known to require a longer time interval after application of the stimulus than sweet or contact. It is natural that time should elapse before actual damage to the cells begins, and that in the meantime other sensations, corresponding to less drastic effects upon the cells, should be felt.

The question must also be very carefully considered whether the immediate conditioning of consciousness can be referred exclusively to the conducting nerve cells. That all pain involves damage to some cells or other seems almost certain, and that it always involves such damage to the receptor cells is at least somewhat probable. As to events at the brain end of the circuit, practically nothing is known. Whether these "jungles of neurology" can ever be illuminated sufficiently to settle the question as to whether or not pain is the consciousness of cellular injury must be left to the future to determine.

### SECTION 39. THE VERIFICATION OF PANPSYCHISM

If the particular sense qualities which we intuit characterize, in this particularity, not so much things in themselves as the biological uses which are made of objects, it may none the less be true that things in themselves must be conceived in terms of a general analogy with the qualities of our experience. The object may not be red or blue or sweet, but there may be something vaguely like these qualities in things, quite apart from human experience. Upon the affective theory, this "may" is equivalent to the statement that panpsychism may be true. .

The principal obstacle to the acceptance of this doctrine—apart from sheer irreligious prejudice—has been the fact that the lower we go in the scale of organic beings the more uncertain does the "inference by analogy" to the feelings, if any, of such creatures become, until it appears to lose all force entirely. It is just here that the conception of an immediate participation in somatic cellular feeling becomes epistemologically important. For it would mean that our knowledge of other sentient individuals came to us in two ways rather than in one, and that at the very point where the inference by analogy approached its weakest stage—in the one-celled animal, a radically different type of evidence, based on direct intuition, entered to strengthen it. Thus panpsychism becomes in principle a doubly verifiable hypothesis. It is well known that two independent arguments for a conclusion are, taken together, strong as the product, and not merely as the sum, of the strengths of each.

Let us suppose that, by tracing the continuous analogy of behavior and structure—in themselves two lines, rather than one, of evidence—by which man is related even to a one-celled creature, some probability, however weak, could be established that under certain circumstances the nerve cells of a man's finger and the therewith-connected conducting fibers and brain cells would undergo suffering, at least if they were sentient at all, and suppose also it could be shown that under the very same conditions the man himself habitually feels pain in the finger, would we not have some real evidence in this coincidence of the two chains of testimony that the inference by analogy was correct?[11] Then if, further, we could satisfy ourselves of the truth of the affective analysis of sensations generally, we should be justified in extending the same treatment to other sensations than that of pain, and in fact would begin to see in all experience a clue to the feeling state of creatures besides ourselves.

It is also noteworthy that even the inference to the feelings of other human beings would be strengthened. For by observing both the macroscopic or bodily and the microscopic or cellular structure and behavior of another, we should have a double clue to his feelings, including the objective feelings constituting his sensations.

It is to be admitted and emphasized that such speculations will amount to very little indeed until they have been given a more specific character. The dimensions of feeling quality as directly given must be traced more definitely than we have succeeded in doing in the preceding chapter, and these dimensions must be correlated with physiological variables, in compatibility with the all-or-none transmission of the nervous impulse. This all-or-none law suggests that we must look for the explanation of qualitative variations exclusively in "modulations" of

---

[11] If the analysis of space given in chap. vi is correct, then the experience of a feeling as spatially distinct from the self, as "there" in the finger, is absolute proof of the existence of a feeling center not identical with the human self. For "depth is epistemological" —to repeat the key phrase of the analysis.

the pattern of pulses, not in the character of the single pulses. The picture developed in this section emphasizes, on the contrary, the quality of feeling in the cellular units. It must, however, be remembered that the law deals directly only with a single dimension—namely, intensity—and while the implication is that the entire character of the nerve action in a given transmission or terminal nerve fiber is independent, except for timing, of the character of the stimulus, we cannot assume that this time pattern itself has no effects of a non-intensive nature upon the nervous process. Yet it is clearly sound procedure to neglect such subtleties until we have made much more progress in unraveling the impulse patterns. Now all pattern as immediately given is subject to aesthetic principles of concord and discord. Perhaps, then, the quality of our experiences depends chiefly not upon that of the cellular units as psychic individuals but upon our sense of the smoothness or other Gestalt qualities of the configurations formed by these units as fused into the oneness of our awareness. On the other hand, by our general panpsychic principle, such Gestalt quality would also enter into the constituent units, so that the two points of view we have just been contrasting are not altogether different. In any case the significant fact is that the physiological aspect of non-intensive dimensions is as yet a nearly complete mystery.[12] Where all theories are so nearly at a complete loss, even such vaguely promising possibilities as those we have been considering may deserve attention. There remains the problem of the inorganic physical realities external to the human body. Here no direct intuition of appreciable vividness is possible; we are reduced to analogy alone for all particularization of the general panpsychistic doctrine. Nevertheless, the possibility of a direct check upon the principle of analogy at a point which we may perhaps term halfway between the higher animals, the indubitably psychical organisms, and the simplest of physical entities, electrons, protons, photons—the point, that is, which is occupied by the cells of the human body—forbids us to declare im-

---

[12] See Troland's masterly discussion of the possibilities (*Psychophysiology* I, 109–28).

possible or fruitless the application of this principle lower down on the scale.[13]

### SECTION 40. CONCLUSION: SOME PREDICTIONS

The theory of the affective continuum implies that whatever qualities exist can be related as values of variables intersecting in the same system. It also implies that qualities of human experience correspond in some degree to qualities of neural and somatic cellular experiences which, by the bond of sympathy which is the psycho-physical relation, form their physiological conditions. The particular form of these general relationships cannot be deduced but must be discovered by observation, and the work of discovery is a task of psychology, not of philosophy. However, the division of labor is not rigid, especially in times of rapid advance. I venture upon the following predictions, which are based not upon any philosophical doctrine alone but upon more or less inadequate factual observations as interpreted by the doctrine of affective continuity.

That pitch is a physiological analogue of visual brightness to a far greater extent than the place theory implied is a prediction which has already been verified. Further work may be required, however, to put this outcome beyond reasonable doubt. I predict that a similar basis for the brightness effect will be found in all senses.

The suggestion that there is such a thing as auditory density has also apparently been confirmed. This means that the brain distinguishes between the number of pulses reaching the entire auditory area (loudness); the number coming over a single fiber or, above seven or eight hundred per second, the number coming over each co-operating fiber pair or triplet (pitch brightness); the percentage of fibers active in a given section (density). This statement, of course, requires refinement and qualification.

The auditory neural response will be found to vary at some

---

[13] It seems necessary frequently to remind the critics of panpsychism that the question is not whether sticks and stones are sentient individuals; for such objects are not individuals except in the sense in which a crowd is so. Indeed, the group mind may well be thought to have a much higher degree of effective individual unity than that swarm of molecules called a "stone."

point in a still further manner, which will prove analogous to the "modulations" or what not which underlie visual chroma.[14] Such variations will in both visual and auditory cases be polar, i.e., with incompatible extremes, and will thus explain complementary neutralization. Pure tones will spiral in terms of these polar contrasts so as to make octaves, except for saturation, duplicates in terms of them,[15] and half-octaves duplicates in one dimension but not in the other. Vowels will be approximately neutral in both dimensions.

Red vision involves some physiological factor which, or something like it, occurs in the feeling of warmth, and green or blue-green has the same relation to the sense of coolness, also (Pikler) to sour taste.

That at least two of the basic odors, sweet and sour, are close analogues of tastes has, as we have seen, been confirmed by practical procedures employed by a group of commercial chemists. Physiological analogues will doubtless be found in due time.

Pleasure will be found to occur under conditions of cellular health, and pain and suffering, of cellular damage—for instance, encroachment upon the refractory period.

The general notion of affective continuity is not dependent upon the complete success of these predictions, but the degree of success which they enjoy will aid in evaluating and, when necessary, in modifying the notion as I have presented it.

Turning from these details, and looking toward the long future of science, one can discern three possibilities: (1) The various natural sciences may never be united in a single science, disclosing fundamental laws valid for all aspects of nature. It needs no argument to show that a scientist would not choose this outcome if he could see any way to avert it. (2) Physics, suitably

[14] See Glen A. Fry, "Modulation of the Optic Nerve-Current as a Basis for Color-Vision," *American Journal of Psychology*, XLV, No. 3 (1933), 488 ff. On the general problem of the neural basis of quality, see Paul Weiss, "Neue experimentelle Beweise für das Resonanzprinzip der Nerventätigkeit," *Biologischer Zentralblatt*, L (1930), 357–72.

[15] For some fascinating physiological possibilities to explain this see Poliak, *Main Afferent Systems in the Cortex* ("University of California Publications in Anatomy," Vol. II [1932]), chap. xii. I owe this reference to Mr. Alvin M. David.

generalized, may absorb biology and psychology, and become the science of nature, of the *physis*, which the Greek founders of science so ardently sought. To most persons it needs little argument to show that the conception of such an outcome is self-contradictory, since the kind of psychology which it implies could not be admitted by any man in his own case, as a complete account of his own nature. The contention that at least it might be the complete account of that in his nature which was capable of scientific treatment simply amounts to saying that a scientific account of nature as a whole is impossible, and thus it should, and however positivists may not like this it will, leave men of science dissatisfied. (3) Psychology, suitably generalized to include all organisms—electrons and all known individuals being so classified—may absorb biology and physics. This psychology will be both behavioristic and introspective, but all the laws will ultimately be statable in introspective terms, since we know and can imagine nothing which cannot be put completely in terms of conceivable experience. Behavior is simply the changing way in which individuals are presented in and influence each other's experience. Nothing inconsistent with this is known.

The first view has never been the chief inspiration of science, except in the negative and provisional sense of enabling physics to dominate the intellectual scene long enough to get itself thoroughly established. As soon as this had taken place, Cartesian dualism began to give way to Spinozistic, Leibnizian, or a modernized Democritean monism, that is, to approximations to views (2) or (3). View (2), in the atomistic form most neatly presented by Lucretius, has haunted scientific men through two thousand years, seldom really convincing them, yet a potent source of intellectual hope and endeavor. In the last few generations, however, it has been impressed upon more and more people that the successes of atomism are not in the least due to the concept of matter, except in its noncommittal meaning of whatever it is that occupies space, but to the pattern of individuation and change which materialism has ascribed to physical nature. Now it is just those features of the pattern which are peculiarly materialistic that physics has rejected. It is impossible to mention, and no one has mentioned, any fact which physics now asserts about the pattern of individual occurrences which contradicts the supposition that individuals as such are sentient creatures. It requires no prophet to see what this means. Leibniz becomes more relevant than Democritus, and a Leibniz freed precisely of those concessions to Democritus which were extracted from him by the materialism of Newtonian science (e.g., the absolute character of its atomic concept, the lack of social give and take, the windowlessness of the materialist's world). The possibility of a single science of nature at once follows. All individuals become comparable to ourselves, and physics may prove to be nothing but the behavioristic side of the psychology or sociology of the most universally distributed and low-grade or simple individuals. This is the only conception that can even pretend to represent an absolute ideal of scientific success. Its advantage is unique, and with every advance of science can only become more apparent. For everything moves toward it—at least in the sense that it brings us nearer to the completion of less ambitious programs, and hence to the time when they can no longer function as goals—and nothing can carry us beyond it.[16]

The reason this ultimate program seems so remote or incredible is partly that we have as yet no real conception of the variables exhibited in human experience, and hence do not see how widely different values from any occurring in our experience are abstractly conceivable as missing areas or extended portions of the domains of potential characters which the variables permit. The reason is also partly our ignorance of the details of nature on its behavioristic side, the superficiality of even our physics and, much more, of our biology and physiology.

When science has gained a more perfect picture of the spatio-temporal patterns exhibited by the life and adventures of a particle, including perhaps the evolution of the cosmos from a stage in which it did not contain this particle, and into one in

[16] The evidence for panpsychism could be adequately stated only in a much more extensive discussion. Such a discussion would include particularly an examination of the categories of time and causality. (I have touched upon these in *The Monist*, 1933, pp. 63–65, and in *The Journal of Philosophy*, XXIX [1932] pp. 364 ff.)

which it will no longer contain it, then perhaps speculations as to an inner life of the particle, its pleasures, displeasures, etc., will take a more definite form. All science may thus become natural history, and all individuals studied by science, fellow-creatures. Physics will be but the most primitive branch of comparative psychology or of general sociology.

This goal may seem fantastically remote. But inasmuch as it is offered as the absolute ideal of scientific achievement, there is no reason why it should not present difficulties. Fifty years ago cultivated adults seem to have been scarcely able to enter into the minds of their own children, or of savages. Savages themselves read their own humanity into animals. To abstract from those subtleties and complexities which distinguish the human from the subhuman mind is one of the most difficult of intellectual feats, and the form which the problem assumes in panpsychism, taken as an interpretation of quantum physics, is a limiting extreme. For this reason it is a misunderstanding to reject the panpsychic program as anthropomorphic, since the attempt is precisely to abstract completely from the specifically human in order to conceive the very lowest of the merely animal modes of feeling.

We think that there is an absolute gulf of emergent novelty between our psychic makeup and the constitution of electrons because we do not see in a systematic way either the lines of variation within our own makeup or the pattern of electronic constitution which is to be reached by projection of those lines to a point short, by some relatively small extent, of their disappearance in nonentity. We do not see the path, or by foreshortening we confuse its ultimate and its penultimate extent. And it is not surprising that we have difficulty also in following the path in the direction away from nonentity to the maximal being which is God. The start in either of these or in any direction must be made in ourselves as a section of the possible variations of existence. The method must be geometry, arithmetic, and the observation of phenomena under laboratory, and other, conditions—including those conditions of imaginative experiment which define the "armchair" method of philosophy.

# APPENDIX A
# THE AFFECTIVE CONTINUUM IN THEOLOGY

Since theology is now passing through its profoundest revolution since the early centuries of the Christian Era, it is impossible that brief reference to it should be free from the danger, if not the certainty, of serious misunderstanding. Nevertheless, the bearings of the concept of affective continuity upon the theistic hypothesis are so unmistakable that some discussion of them may be appropriate. It must, however, be definitely understood that I do not believe that the revolution referred to can ever be undone, and that I have no interest in giving any encouragement to the groups who are trying to lead us back to the methods and results of medieval theology. These methods are non-relative, non-quantitative, non-dimensional, and hence opposed to the notion of method which has been stressed in this book; and in their results the popular quantitative notions of all-knowing, all-controlling, at-all-times-existing, etc., are subordinated to technical conceptions such as absolute, immutable, timeless, *ens a se*, *totum simul*, which are held to be more exact, but which, in my judgment, should not be so estimated by anyone with much understanding of modern logic. I also entirely fail to find in them a plausible referent of religious experiences.

Some years ago there appeared in a prominent magazine an excellent account of the inseparability, in the writer's personal experience, of the nominally quite distinct experiences of light and spiritual exaltation.[1] The inseparability appeared as a kind of identity, which the subject found mysterious enough from the standpoint of her scientific gleanings, but stubbornly inescapable as an experiential fact. Subsequently she learned that it was a commonplace of religious and mystical literature, a universal truism indeed, that the Divine appears literally as an inward light. Moreover, one should not forget the constant use of every variety of sense metaphor to characterize the Divine Presence. If even the ordinary worshiper were deprived of the "radiance," the "warmth"—nay, with minds not enslaved to silly aesthetic snobberies, even the "sweetness" and the "fragrance"—of the vision beatific, he would find his capacity for expression seriously impoverished.

Theological theory has not altogether failed to take account of these facts of experience, and certainly the logic of the theological tenet implies that sensory qualities must be regarded as possessing spiritual content. Both in Occident and in Orient this view may be found; and the grounds for it on the logical side are so obvious that I can only regard it as an instance of the illogicality of mankind that it has not been far more commonly accepted by religious think-

---

[1] See Jane Steger, "Some Notes on Light," *Atlantic Monthly*, CXXXVIII (1926), 315–25.

ers than history shows it to have been. For if one is a thoroughgoing believer in an ultimate Divinity, a spiritual Creator, or omnipresent Life, one is obliged to hold that this Divinity is somehow manifested everywhere, that the Creator is expressed in some degree in his creation, in all that is. Strictly regarded, the statement that man is made in his maker's image cannot be taken to ascribe more than a relative distinction to man among the creatures, for in some degree the statement must be true of all created things as such. In the Middle Ages it was indeed a commonplace that all things partake of being just in so far as they bear some resemblance to the Divine Being who in some sense is Being itself.[2] To be wholly unlike God is to be wholly unlike being, to be pure non-being or nothing. Now God is not a composite of parts, such that a man could resemble him in respect to one of these parts and not to others. Resemblance must be to his nature as a whole. Hence if we say God is perfect spirit, then whatever spirit may mean, all things must partake, in some degree, of spirituality. And if God is infinite love, then all things must possess and embody love, in however slight or embryonic a form.

It requires no exceptional mental power to deduce the affective continuum as a corollary. The inductive verification of affective continuity may not establish the truth of theology, but (unless there is a flaw in the foregoing reasoning) its inductive refutation would establish the falsity of the only theology that is religiously significant and logically definite.[3]

[2] Aquinas said: "The essence of God is the perfect resemblance of all things, for it is their universal principle."

[3] This theology is the subject of a projected book, *The New Vision of God*, and of an article to appear in *The New Humanist* (1934), "Philosophy's New Alternative to Scholasticism."

# APPENDIX B

# WHY THE CURRENT DOCTRINE OF PITCH AND LOUDNESS AROSE

The criticism of an almost universally accepted doctrine is greatly strengthened when the critic is able to explain in a reasonable way the prevalence of that doctrine. For the prevalence of the non-intensive notion of pitch there are a number of possible causes. Some of these have been sufficiently indicated in section 6, but there are others.

The first is that it is usually of more practical importance to note pitch and total intensity (the resultant of pitch and volume) than to distinguish volume as a separate aspect. For volume, unlike the area of colors, has no direct counterpart in the environment. Its chief importance is as a dimension of intensity. This is doubtless why many practical workers in acoustics suppose "volume" to be a mere synonym for "loudness," an error to be balanced against the opposite extreme of holding it to be a mere function of pitch. But anyone who compares a very loud note with a very soft one an octave or two below will discover that the volume relationship of the two conforms to neither formula.

A second cause of confusion lies in the fact that in vision brightness or intensity is determined by the energy rather than the frequency of the stimulus, whereas in audition pitch is a pure function of frequency. But the all-or-none law, together with the discovery that visual intensity is neurologically a matter of frequency, removes this discrepancy between the two brightnesses.

Third, that low sounds are feebler as well as "darker," that these two designations are the same, would presumably have been seen by more persons were it not that, as Boring has pointed out, the connection between volume and intensity has been seriously confused in the past by the failure to vary the stimulus in one way only at a time; for, in experiments where frequency was varied, the same physical energy was used throughout, which meant that the amplitude increased with descending pitch. The conclusion drawn—volume is a function of frequency—was thus, as Boring says, "an artifact of the experiments." That volume is at least partly a matter of amplitude can be demonstrated in a few seconds at the piano, where the same note struck, now softly, now loudly, varies unmistakably in size.

The fourth, and perhaps the most important, cause of the failure to analyze loudness into volume and pitch lies in the complexity introduced into this analysis by the overtones. Low notes, as ordinarily heard, are low notes plus high notes, the addition increasing the average intensity (though not as a rule sufficiently to change the intensity of the major portion of the volume, i.e., to raise the apparent pitch—though this may happen); and thus the feebleness of the low notes in themselves is not always noticed.

A fifth confusion arises from a misreading of the relations of "brightness" to "sharpness," or of "dulness" to "bluntness." Sharpness is the effect of intensity plus narrow or clearly defined outline. Now of course, given greater intensity, both reduced quantity and increased distinctness of volumic outline become perceptually possible. Hence high notes which are normally small and always intense are also "pointed" or sharp, and low notes are blunt. This has led some to suppose that the brightness of high notes is their volumic character (Watt). Then there is the aspect of clearness ("clear as a bell"). This term is somewhat ambiguous. It seems to mean clearness and distinctness and singleness of quality as contrasted with a confused qualitative mixture. Here again high notes tend to be clearer, partly because they are freer from overtones, partly because they are temporally steadier, and finally because they are more intense. The dependence of distinctness upon intensity leads to the use of "clear" to denote ambiguously either. French *clair* applied to vision is also ambiguous in this fashion. Remembering finally that variations in brightness sometimes occur, or at least are held to do so, within the same pitch,[1] and especially in connection with the blurred character of vowel sounds, we will not be surprised to find the theory put forth that brightness is due to the "saliency," i.e., the striking distinctness of the pitch effect.[2] This is like saying that a spider's web is sharp because it is thin, whereas the truth is that sharpness implies firmness, i.e., strength, as well as thinness. A bright color can, against the proper background, be salient because it is bright, i.e., intense; but the brightness is not the clarity of outline or the distinctness of quality, but the presupposition of these.[3] Again a "sharp" or "acute" pain is surely an intense one; why should "sharp" in the musical sense (as opposed to "flat") be made, like musical brightness, such an absolute exception? As for the alleged independent variability of brightness and pitch, has it really been proved? For pure tones admittedly not; on the contrary.[4] With vowels, when the bluntness is distinguished from the brightness, as it logically should be, the identity of pitch and brightness may perhaps still not be unambiguously clear, but it must be remembered that the admitted pitch complexity of vowels renders the pitch judgment itself a trifle ambiguous. It appears to denote the mean pitch, i.e., on the brightness theory, the mean brightness or intensity. Now in thinking of bright colors, and of normal high tones, we naturally expect a relatively uniform, clearly outlined intensity. The necessity for assessing a brightness

[1] R. M. Ogden, *Hearing* (London, 1924), pp. 59–62. As Professor Ogden has kindly informed me, this passage does not express his present views.

[2] *Ibid.*, pp. 94–98; also L. T. Troland, *Psychophysiology*, II, 223 f., 358; I, 271.

[3] Professor Ogden himself points out (p. 154) that high notes are "intrinsically more intensive." This shows clearly that it is putting the cart before the horse to explain the brightness of high notes by their pointedness. For then their intensity becomes inexplicable; whereas if we identify intensity, brightness, and pitch, the pointedness and other aspects may all be explained in the simplest possible manner. Troland's view has similar implications. His nerve-frequency theory of pitch implies that the latter is brightness because it is intensity.

[4] G. J. Rich, "A Study of Tonal Attributes," *American Journal of Psychology*, XXX (1919), 121–64; also Troland, *op. cit.*, I, 271.

mean may thus somewhat mislead the brightness judgment. But the broad fact stands out that vowels vary in brightness not chiefly as their pitch uniformity but as their mean pitch altitude varies. Nor have I seen any careful presentation of the evidence for the statement that a vowel is less bright than a tone of the "same" pitch. That there is something less vivid—or, as one would say with colors, less saturated—about it seems to me so; but this involves perhaps a loss of octave quality, which, if one admits it at all, is clearly not brightness. That the vowel is less "clear" or distinct is also evident; but a distinct sound is no more the same as a bright one than a distinct color is the same as a bright one.

Again, there is the evidence from the siren whistle as employed in Abraham's and other experiments.[5] Here it is shown that brightness varies widely while frequency and pitch remain constant. But this pitch constancy is by no means unqualified, a fact which renders questionable the interpretations of Ogden and Troland,[6] who, partly on the basis of this constancy, treat brightness as an attribute independent of pitch height. My respect for, as well as immense indebtedness to, these authors notwithstanding, the facts force me to conclude and the importance of the question leads me to point out that the phenomena discovered by Abraham call for a quite different interpretation. Abraham proved that the length of each wave-trough, and not merely the wave-frequency per second, exercised an effect upon the sound heard. This held for two cases: (a) where but a single wave, and hence no frequency at all, constituted the source of the sound; and (b) where the frequency determined the fundamental tone, but the "primary wave," or individual wave-thickness, determined the brightness. In (a) wide differences of pitch were produced by differences in the primary wave. In (b) Abraham shows that wide differences in the intensities of the partials, whose presence was manifest, were the basis of the brightness variations, and further that these partials could not possibly be explained exclusively as overtones according to the Fourrier analysis of the frequency tone, but involved also partial tones produced by the primary wave. But that the brightness arose from variations in the relative strengths of partials of various pitches Abraham nowhere questions but everywhere insists upon.[7] If we assume the brightness or intensity theory of pitch, these facts all fall into place readily enough. The dominant pitch (intensity) is the most voluminous, forming thus the main mass of the sound. The higher

[5] O. Abraham, "Zur physiologischen Akustik von Wellenlänge und Schwingungszahl," *Zeitschrift für Sinnesphysiologie*, LI (1920), 121–52.

[6] Ogden, *op. cit.*, pp. 59–62, 93–94; Troland, *op. cit.*, p. 223. In both of these works there is an error in the references to Abraham's paper (Vol. L instead of Vol. LI).

[7] See also Ogden, *op. cit.*, pp. 60–61, 93–94. Even without going behind this author's account of Abraham's work one cannot but question his interpretation. Troland likewise summarizes Abraham's result as showing that brightness is a matter not of frequency or pitch alone but of "frequency composition." This seems verbally the position we are defending. Yet in the same breath Troland rejects the pitch theory of brightness and in his final account of this character relies primarily not upon frequency composition but upon phase discrepancies internal to a single frequency (the "bending" of the neural wave) (see Troland, *loc. cit.*).

and thinner partials vary in intensity, but as pitch is intensity, variations in relative strengths of different partials can only mean variations in their relative volumes. Each higher partial is an area of brightness—the brighter the higher the pitch. The total brightness effect depends accordingly in part upon the extent of the bright areas within the darker background of the more massive dominant tone. Therefore, the more numerous and voluminous the higher tones, the brighter the sound mass as a whole. Finally, and this renders the evidence almost all that could be desired, the brighter sounds in (*b*) were in fact produced by the very conditions which in (*a*) gave rise to a noise of higher pitch (namely, small holes or a peripheral position of the holes causing a short primary wave). Hence we may infer that in (*b*) the bright sounds owed this brightness to partials of high pitch caused by the character of the primary wave. There is accordingly nothing in Abraham's work to necessitate or even to suggest the separation of brightness as an introspective attribute from pitch and volume. Nor is this Abraham's point, which is rather that the composition of pitches and volumes is determined not solely by frequency and amplitude but also by wave-thickness—in short, a psycho-physical, not a psychological, contention. Inasmuch, too, as the brightness variations in question were accompanied by marked vowel character, the supposed non-identity of pitch and brightness alleged for vowels may also be regarded as discredited by these same experiments.[8]

A very important obstacle—the last which we have to consider—to the understanding of auditory brightness has been that even in vision it is far from obvious that brightness and intensity coincide. Yet, as Pikler has observed, the relation between the sensation of black and the tendency to fall asleep, in contrast to the wakefulness induced by white,[9] affords evidence of this coincidence sufficient at least to make us critical of the arguments used in support of its denial.[10]

---

[8] Jaensch has shown how widely different vowel characters can be made to appear at the same pitch (through an identical fundamental tone), although the vowel character itself is determined by "formants" at widely differing pitches. This confirms the supposition that in Abraham's experiment the brightness-vowel variations were variations in the pitch of the formants (Jaensch, *op. cit.*, pp. 64-68).

[9] This is one more illustration of the possibility of describing quality through its internal relations (see sec. 4) with behavior.

[10] For a view somewhat similar to Pikler's see James Ward, "Is 'Black' a Sensation?" *British Journal of Psychology*, I, 407-27.

# APPENDIX C
# BRIGHTNESS AS A UNIVERSAL ATTRIBUTE

The identity of brightness as an introspective variable has been checked experimentally by Hornbostel. His subjects compared a certain sensation $a$ with a sensation $b$ taken from another sense, and compared $b$ with a sensation $c$ taken from a third sense. Finally, $a$ and $c$ were compared. When $a$ and $b$ were judged equal in brightness, and likewise $b$ and $c$, then $a$ and $c$ also were found equally bright.[1] Evidence appearing to discredit these results has, however, recently been obtained at Harvard by Cohen. It was found that the judgment of degree of brightness varied in that if the sensation from one sense was one of a group of sensations from that sense it was judged medium bright, very bright, or dull, according to its position in the group, and its equality in brightness with a sensation from another sense varied accordingly. It is a question if this work proves anything more than that the matter of brightness equality is not so easily settled as Hornbostel thought. One fact at least is not put in doubt: the direction of greater or less brightness is the same for all observers and for all conditions.[2]

[1] See E. M. von Hornbostel in Flueger, *Archive für gesamte Physiologie*, CCXXVII, 517 f.

[2] See Nathan E. Cohen, "Equivalence of Brightness across Modalities," *American Journal of Psychology*, January, 1934, pp. 117-19.

# APPENDIX D

## GOETHE'S *FARBENLEHRE*

In the history of sensory theory the work of Goethe on colors occupies a special and rather puzzling position. Nothing, indeed, is more singular, in the life of this singular man, than his theory of colors and its destiny. Intended by the great poet and distinguished scientist as a contribution to science, it found favor only among philosophers, and then not chiefly among those primarily interested in science. Regarded by its originator with truculent pride as among his greatest achievements and chief titles to fame, it has been treated by so fair-minded a critic as Helmholtz as, in the main, an extraordinary blunder, based upon a misapprehension of the nature of science. To the physicist, an absurd heresy; to the psychologist, a mixture of incidentally interesting details with essentially false or trivial first principles; to the biographer, a rather embarrassingly inconsequential chapter—considering its bulk—in the renowned man's life-work. It almost recalls Bishop Berkeley's tar-water! Is this, then, the whole truth of the matter?

Let us first note that it was not in the nature of things that Goethe's theory of colors should have been understood, either by his contemporaries or even by many of his successors. It was Goethe's aim that his conceptions should have as empirical a foundation as those of any natural science; but, unfortunately, this ambition was combined with a way of thinking which must immediately alienate the scientifically trained, and confuse the philosophical of our day (who have adopted the standpoint of science). The peculiarity of this way of thinking is seen in Goethe's resolute refusal to admit, and inability to perceive, any basic distinction between physics and psychology. For him, the real physical world is the world as we experience it, and thus the external causes of our sensations of color will not differ essentially from the qualities of color given in the sensations themselves. This, of course, appears to be in plain contradiction with the results of Newtonian physics. The violent polemic against Newton scattered throughout the *Farbenlehre* is accordingly easily understood. The analysis of light into essentially invisible colorless particles was a monstrosity to one who held that the essential factors of nature must be capable of directly revealing themselves. Now although it is true that contemporary theories of scientific method, with their reactions against the "bifurcation of nature," mere atomism, and the rest of the dogmatic metaphysics of earlier science, render Goethe's position decidedly more intelligible from the scientific standpoint than it could have been to the older orthodox attitude, nevertheless, it cannot be said that the progress of physical science has resulted in the victory of the Goethean as against the Newtonian view of light and color. The analytic-particle view of light, and of nature generally, is still with us, and shows no sign of abandoning the field. If we, then, grant that Goethe's problem was—as he himself maintained—none other than that of Newton, it must be confessed that his solution was hopelessly erroneous. So, with the exception of a few discredited philosophers, the critics have concluded.

# APPENDIX

But may it not be that, confused in Goethe's mind with the physical problem, was involved one of quite different type, say a phenomenological one, and may not Goethe's solution, as an answer to this problem, possess something of the truth and importance he claimed for his theory as a whole? The fact that he supposed that a description of color data as immediately given would yield at the same time a physical explanation of these phenomena does not necessarily prove the entire falsity of his descriptions.

What, then, was the upshot of Goethe's theory of colors as a description or phenomenology? Two principles, he held, were involved in color vision, as indeed in all experience and in all nature. One of these, positive in character, is illustrated in its purest form by white light; the other, essentially negative, by darkness. Colors in general arise from the varying degrees of predominance of one or the other of these two factors. Thus yellow is highly positive and akin to light; blue, relatively negative and akin to darkness. The point of greatest difficulty is to see how two dimensions are to be conjured out of what seems but a single contrast of positive and negative. However this difficulty is to be met, it is worth noting that the characterizations of color as active or passive, positive or negative, warm or cold, and the like were based in Goethe's case upon probably the most adequate observational evidence ever brought to bear upon the question prior to the twentieth century. That Goethe's method, whatever its limitations of principle, was applied with great skill and thoroughness, and in a truly scientific spirit, has been authoritatively recognized by Helmholtz.

The great fact in nature, according to Goethe, was the fact of polar opposition, subject to the condition of organic interdependence. In terms of such categories his color theory was conceived, and its merit is shown not only by its agreement, in so far, with the physics of a century later (to which electrical polarity is basic) but also by the verifiable relevance of his descriptions of color phenomena—for instance, his excellent account of color harmony, in which sphere his work has not gone altogether unrecognized. The fact alone that Goethe conceived the problem of colors as essentially the problem of nature as given to one sense, as essentially an integral phase of the philosophy and science of nature, whereas to the introspective psychologist red is "just red," with no more of nature, in any intelligible sense, in its essence than there might be in a Thomistic angel—rather less—is enough to give importance to the Goethean doctrine. Goethe's assumption was that, as Chief Justice Holmes has it, "nature is all of a piece," and there is nothing so mean (or ineffable) that we may not see in it the universal laws. It follows that even a "simple" quality of color contains somehow in itself the world-energies, and since the color is nothing if not something to be seen, this universal content of the color must be capable of being seen in it. The future of the theory of sensation lies—as the whole shift of our times away from the self-contained solipsistic view of consciousness indicates—in the direction of such a view of sense experience as "organic to nature."

Future biographers of Goethe, coming to the chapter of color, may find themselves less embarrassed.[1]

[1] For an attempt to revive and develop Goethe's point of view see Hedwig Conrad-Martius, "Farben," *Jahrbuch für Philosophie und phänomenologische Forschung*, ed. Edmund Husserl (Halle: Max Niemeyer, 1929).

# APPENDIX E

## BIBLIOGRAPHICAL NOTE

There are comparatively few works dealing exclusively with the topic of sensation. Of those written by psychologists, the following are important:

TROLAND, L. T. *Sensation* (Vol. II of his *Principles of Psychophysiology*). New York: Van Nostrand, 1930.

BORING, E. G. *The Physical Dimensions of Consciousness*. New York: Century Co., 1933.

PIKLER, JULIUS. *Schriften zur Anpassungstheorie des Empfindungsvorganges*. Leipzig: JOHANN AMBROSIUS BARTH.
- No. 1. *Hypothesenfreie Theorie der Gegenfarben*. 1919. Pp. 104.
- No. 2. *Theorie der Konsonanz und Dissonanz*. 1920. Pp. 34.
- No. 3. *Theorie der Empfindungstärke und insbesondere des Weberschen Gesetzes*. 1920. Pp. 26.
- No. 4. *Theorie der Empfindungsqualität als Abbild des Reizes*. 1922. Pp. 107.
- No. 5. *Theorie des Gedächtnisses*. 1927. Pp. 43.

On the physiological side E. D. Adrian's *The Basis of Sensation* (New York: W. W. Norton, 1928) is a classic. It is to be supplemented by his *The Mechanism of Nervous Action: Electrical Studies of the Neurone* (Oxford Press and University of Pennsylvania Press, 1932). Johannes von Kries's *Allgemeine Sinnesphysiologie* (Leipzig, 1923), although antiquated, contains valuable material.

There are a number of works devoted to the physiology and psychology of a single sense or group of senses. Some of these are:

HELMHOLTZ, H. *Physiological Optics*. trans. from the third German ed. Optical Society of America, 1924.

LADD-FRANKLIN, C. *Colour and Colour Theories*. New York: Harcourt, Brace & Co., 1929.

HOUSTON, R. A. *Vision and Colour Vision*. London, New York, and Toronto: Longmans, Green & Co., 1932.

STUMPF, K. *Tonpsychologie*. Leipzig, 1883-90.

OGDEN, R. M. *Hearing*. New York: Harcourt, Brace & Co., 1924.

JAENSCH, E. R. *Grundfragen der Akustik und Tonpsychologie*. Leipzig, 1929.

HENNING, H. *Der Geruch*. Leipzig, 1916.

PARKER, G. H. *Smell, Taste, and Allied Senses in the Vertebrates*. Philadelphia and London: Lippincott, 1922.

# APPENDIX

By philosophers the following books have appeared:

LAVELLE, L. *La dialectique du monde sensible.* Strasbourg: Imprimerie Alsacienne, 1921.
FLESSNER, H. *Die Einheit der Sinne.* Bonn: Friedrich Cohen, 1923.
PRICE, H. H. *Perception.* London: Methuen, 1932.

All of these have value, but in none of them is there much reference to experimental data. Also there is little explicit treatment of the emotional theory of sense perception. This is particularly true of the last-mentioned work, which, though in many respects a most excellent study, totally ignores this theory, in spite of its increasing importance in philosophy.

The profoundest analysis of sensation in its most general character which anyone has yet published is, in my opinion, to be found in the writings of A. N. Whitehead, especially in *Adventures of Ideas* ([New York: Macmillan, 1933], pp. 225–29, 274–77, 334), *Process and Reality* ([New York: Macmillan, 1929], Part II, chap. iv), and *Symbolism, Its Meaning and Effect* ([New York: Macmillan, 1927], pp. 13–29). No use is made by Whitehead of definite experimental data.

Two writers who have tried to combine the detailed or experimental and the more general or philosophical aspects of the sensory problem are:

BRENTANO, FRANZ. *Untersuchungen zur Sinnespsychologie.* Leipzig: Duncker & Humblot, 1907.
REISER, O. L. *The Alchemy of Light and Color.* New York: Norton, 1928.

Brentano is a mixture of brilliant insights (including some not easily found elsewhere) and special pleadings. Reiser's little book is slight but suggestive.

The following is a list of my own previous publications having for their joint subject the philosophy and psychology of sensation:

"Sense Quality and Feeling Tone", *Proceedings of the Seventh International Congress of Philosophy, at Oxford*, pp. 168–72.
"Ethics and the Assumption of Purely Private Pleasures," *International Journal of Ethics*, XL, 496–515, esp. 502–4, 507.
"The Intelligibility of Sensations," *Monist*, 1934.
See also *ibid.*, January, 1933, pp. 65 ff.; *Philosophical Review*, XXXVIII, 289–90.

In a different category from any of the writings yet mentioned is Othmar Reich's *Das Qualitätsproblem der Psychologie und seine Lösung* (Prague, 1933). Originally a musician and composer, the author was led by contradictions between musical experience and traditional psychological theory (represented, e.g., by Stumpf) to investigate the psychology of sensory quality. His conclusion is similar to that of Pikler and to my own (sec. 38); sensation is evaluational in essence and evolves from the organism's feeling of its adaptational relations to its environment. This is also Whitehead's view. Lavelle, the only other author above mentioned who seeks to explain qualities, is an intellectualist-theologian with only slight appreciation of the concrete biological aspects and the rôle of affective tone. But there would be no need for him to deny these factors—indeed strong reasons for his accepting them—so that the works of Pikler, Lavelle, Reich, and Whitehead may all be regarded as pointing to an emotional theory of sense qualities.

The emotional individuality of sense qualities is attested, in respect to one sense, by an astonishingly large literature. I refer to the many books dealing with what Goethe called *die sinnlich-sittliche Wirkungen*, the sensory-spiritual effects, of colors. These books are generally a blend of vivid impressionistic description with more or less fanciful theosophical speculations. Such is Ellen Conroy's *The Symbolism of Colour* (London: William Rider & Son, 1921). A sober and extensive account of the spiritual phases of color experience is Walter Koch's *Psychologische Farbenlehre: Die sinnlich-sittliche Wirkung der Farben* (Halle a.S., 1931). Koch's summary (p. 77) of the *Farben-Urgefühle*—"for yellow a joyous, for blue a serious, for red an excited, for green a calm, and for the mixed colors corresponding mixed feelings"—could be substantially duplicated from almost any of the other books on this subject. His description (p. 232) of black—"the positive destruction of all joy in life and light," "the palpable presence of hopeless nothing," "like an eternal silence without future and without hope," "immovable like a corpse"—forms an interesting and by Koch unnoted contrast to the standard psychological contention that the sensation of black is "as positive" as any other. It appears that those who have studied colors descriptively have not been concerned to apply the descriptive facts to the solution of theoretical problems. As a final reference in color aesthetics, Kandinsky's *Das Geistige in der Kunst* (out of print) may be mentioned as an artist's analysis of the subject.

# INDEX

Abercrombie, 91 n., 153, 159, 182 n.
Abraham, 275–76
Abstraction, 29
   extensive, 25
Activity, 195
   -passivity, 224
Adaptation and qualities, 6, 8, 15, 33, 146 ff., 250 ff.
Adrian, 69, 280
Aesthetic experience, 153
   appreciation, 189
   taste, 185
Aesthetics, 28, 159 ff.
Affection, 9, 99, 115, 129, 130, 134
Affective continuum, the, 9, 36, 108, 116, 126, 200 ff., 266, 271
   tone, 7, 54
All-or-none law, the, 72, 150, 264
Allen, B., 131 n., 196 n.
Allesch, von, 119–20, 122
Analogies between the senses, 68, 74
Analysis, 24, 26, 178
Animals, 112, 245, 257, 259, 261
Animism, 106, 116
Anti-idealism, 106
Antimaterialism, 14
Aquinas, 272 n.
Aristotle, 146, 178, 214
Art, 160, 169
Artists, 182–83
Associations, 137, 169–75, 187–89, 252
Attention, 160, 185
   and feeling, 131 ff.
Atomic analysis, 140, 143–44
Atomism, 4, 11, 268
   in psychology, 138 ff., 209
   relative, 12, 143
Atoms, 14, 17, 25
Audition, 64
Auslander, 74, 75

Awareness, 54, 88, 93, 104, 108, 111, 114, 194, 200–203

Banister, 66 n.
Basch, 182 n.
Beauty, 175, 205
Beebe-Center, 130 n., 131 n., 133 n., 134 n., 156 n., 165 n., 251
Behavior, 152 ff., 268
   and qualities, 27 ff., 196, 244
Behaviorism, 108, 154
Being, 125
Berkeley, 17, 19, 91–94, 182
Bichowsky, 76, 135
Bitter, 146
Black, 21, 58, 64, 148, 184, 212–13, 225, 253, 276
   and white, 209
Blue, 8, 88 n., 148, 219, 253, 255
Boring, 67 n., 70, 71 n., 151 n.
Bosanquet, 88–90, 182 n.
Bradley, 12, 21
Brentano, 138–39, 220, 223, 227, 232 n., 260
Brightness, 31, 59, 61, 65 n., 69, 72, 73 n., 74, 75 n., 128–29, 216, 230, 231, 236, 243, 266
   and pitch, 274 ff.
Brilliance, 211
Broglie, De, 15
Brown, 79, 119
Bullough, 60 n.
Burnett and Dallenbach, 50 n., 77 n.
Burroughs, 83

Cadence, 65
Carritt, 181
Cassirer, 104
Cattell, 136 n.
Cells, 112, 244 ff., 260, 262, 264
Characters, 117–24, 132, 171

283

Chinese, the, 170–71
Classifications in science, 37
Cohen, M. R., 244 n.
Cohen, N., 277
Coherence, aesthetic, 163, 167
Cold, 204
Color, 27, 30, 43, 98, 119, 122, 151, 170, 183, 199, 209 ff., 224, 278 f.
  Cartesian co-ordinates of, 44
  continuum, the, 42, 46–48, 207
  geometry of, 40 ff.
  harmony, 164, 166, 222, 224
  metrical aspects of, 46
  ordinal aspects of, 46
Colored hearing, 65 n., 77, 81, 82
Colors, 60, 62, 165, 184
  characters of, 117–18, 121, 170, 183, 234, 253
  circle of, 166, 221
  complementary, 211, 221
  distance between, 47
  mixture of, 223
  primary, 214 ff., 221
  and sounds, 67, 75, 206, 231, 234
  square of, 47
  surface, 203 n., 231
Common sense, 69, 74, 157, 200
Conrad-Martius, 279 n.
Conroy, 282
Consciousness, 109, 110 n., 113, 201
Content forms, 203
Continuity, 6, 10, 15, 25, 34, 42, 50, 95, 207
Coster, 54
Cries, animal, 259
Croce, 91, 162 n., 169, 180–82
Crocker and Henderson, 239 n.
Cultural theory, the, 172
Cutsworth, 82–83

Dallenbach, 50 n., 77 n.
Darwin, 152
Dashiell, 116
Davis, 71
Democritus, 269
Density of sounds, 64
Depth, 197, 264 n.,

Determinism, 12, 16
Dimmick, 67 n., 210–11
Discontinuity, 7, 10, 12, 15, 34 ff., 57, 59
Diversity, 36
Drake, 144 n.
Dwelshauvers, 136 n.

*Einfühlung*, 182 n.
Emergence, 8, 34, 207
Emotion, 7, 114, 124, 168
Essence, 21, 23
Experience, 8, 190 f.
Expression, 162, 169, 178

Faculty psychology, 137
Faraday's principle, 193
*Farbenlehre*, Goethe's, 278
Fear, 174
Feeling, 7, 14, 38–39, 53, 96, 118, 163, 168, 171, 175, 205
  in cells, 245
  of feeling, 198, 208
  objective, 98, 117 ff., 129
  social, 193
  tone, 52, 111, 179
  and sensation, 37, 50, 116, 122–24, 127, 129, 130, 134
Feelings
  as dimensions of sensory quality, 126, 129
  multi-dimensional view of, 130 n.
  subjective, 126 ff., 179–80, 186
Formalism, 178
Fry, 267
Fundamental conceptions, 6
  traits of mind, 36
Funeral ceremonies, 170
Fusion of sensations, 76

Gestalt psychology, 154, 156
  quality, 265
Goethe, 146, 214, 278
Goldstein, 217
Gray, 68, 77 n., 139, 210
Green, 8, 41, 46, 80, 119, 148, 216–18, 253, 254
  defined, 221
Grudin, 182 n.
Gustatory tetrahedron, the, 237

# INDEX

Haldane, 243
Halverson, 63
Hanslick, 178
Harlow and Stagner, 131 n., 196 n.
Harmony, 164–67, 225–26
Hearing, 257 ff.
  and vision, 228
Heat and pain, 29, 50
Hecht, 67
Hegel, 182
Heimholtz, 6, 30, 77, 84, 278
Henning, 134 n., 237–39, 261
Heterogeneity, sensuous, 77, 80
Hoffman, 239 n.
Hoffman, E. T. W. (the composer), 80 n.
Hogben, 74
Hornbostel, E. M. von, 20, 65 n., 68, 75 n., 80 n., 117 n., 277
Huber, 65 n., 117 n., 120 n.
Huxley, A., 75
Hyletic sensationalism, 90

Idealism, 18, 20, 87–89, 98, 101
  criticism of, 95–99
Idealists, 32, 90, 95, 103
  and realists, 96
Illusions, 124, 175
Imagination, 20
Immanence, 175
Immediacy, 155
Immediate knowledge, 246–47
Incomparability, doctrine of, 80
Indefiniteness, 207
Individuality, idea of, 100
Inexplicables, doctrine of, 26
Inherence, theory of, 177
Intensity, 62, 75, 212, 224, 225, 243
  and brightness, 31, 128
Interest, 99, 102–3
Intermediaries, 201–2
Introspection, 52, 74, 108, 120, 143, 155
Intuition, 37

Jaensch, 136, 229, 276 n.
Joy, 202
Juhasz, 240 n.

Kandinsky, 282
Kiesow, 130 n., 237 n.
King, C. D., 1 n., 131 n., 150, 244
Knight, L., 50 n.
Knowing, feeling, and willing, 36
Koch, 282
Köhler, 80, 156 n.
Kries, von, 140 n., 280
Külpe, 133 n.

Ladd-Franklin, 213
Lavelle, 281
Lear, 52
Leibniz, 66, 93, 94, 95, 106, 143, 181, 190, 269
Leon, 160 n.
Lewis, 12 n., 24, 26, 27, 56
Lipps, 182 n.
Locke, 59 n., 94
Loudness, 61, 63, 66 n., 273
  of colors, 61
Love, 13, 208
Lovejoy, 18 n.

MacDougall, R., 154
Marston, W. M. and E. H., 1, 131 n., 244 n.
Materialism, 11, 13 ff., 20, 90, 101, 181
Matter, 12, 15–18, 90, 102
McDougall, W., 110
Meaning, 118, 185
Melody, 182
Memory, 206
Metaphors, 58, 73
Metaphysics, 4
Miller, D. S., 99 n.
Mind, 39, 100, 155
Minor scale, 172 n.
Mixture conception of secondary colors, 42, 139, 209
Modes, doctrine of, 6, 30 n., 57, 76, 78–81, 83
Monism, aesthetic, 182 n.
Moore, 87–89, 100, 110
Moos, 182 n.

Motive, 113
Mozart, 160 n.
Müller-Freienfels, 130 n.
Music, 171-72, 178, 183, 186, 188, 233
Musical discords, 171
Myers, 81, 187 n.
Mythologies, 104

Nafe, 30, 55 n., 64, 68 n., 75 n., 126, 128-29, 142, 235, 236, 259
Nearness, 196
Negatives, 58
Negativity, 205
Nerves, 247-48
Nervous system, the, 243
Neural frequency, 69-72
Newton, 278
*Niveau*, the, 119, 122
Noises, 229

Objective relativism, 18 n.
Observers, 121-22
Octave quality, 68, 166, 225-26, 228-34
Odors, 60, 236, 238-41, 261-62, 267
Oeser, 133 n.
Ogden, C. K., 112 n., 162 n.
Ogden, R. M., 65 n., 274 n.
Ohm's law, 228, 230
Orange, 41, 43, 79, 80, 119, 147
Order, 163
Overtones, 63, 232
Ozenfant, 170, 171, 183

Paget, R., 230 n.
Pain, 49-58, 94, 129, 202, 234-36, 260 262-63, 267
Panpsychism, 31, 105, 145, 244, 250, 263 ff., 266 n., 269-70
Parker, D. H., 175
Parker, G. H., 111
Pattern, 182 ff., 265
Peirce, 9, 34, 37, 190, 208, 243
Perry, 96, 99
Personality and sensory quality, 32

Phelan, 136 n.
Philosophers, 102, 106, 190, 192
Philosophy, 191
Physics, 15, 16, 145, 157, 190, 267, 269
 of the nervous system, 35
Physiology, 73
Piaget, 105
Pikler, 1 n., 35 n., 50 n., 145 n., 146 ff. 213, 214, 235, 237-40, 261, 276
Pitch, 59, 60, 63, 65, 67, 69-71, 74, 149, 266, 273 ff.
Place theory, the, 69-73
Plates I, 44; II, 221
Plato, 178, 190
Pleasantness, 205
 -unpleasantness, 99, 126-30 n., 133
Pleasure and pain, 94, 202, 262, 267
Plenum of colors, the, 122 ff.
Plurality of attributes, doctrine of, 31
Polarity, 134-35
Poliak, 267 n.
Pragmatism, 156
Pratt, C., 60, 80 n.
Pre-sensation, 76, 135-36, 231
Pressure, 127
Price, H. H., 206 n., 281
Projection theory, the, 1:8
Psychoanalysis, 156
Psychologists, 192
Psychology, 136, 145, 164, 266, 268
 Gestalt, 154, 156, 199
 integrative, 150
 method of, 153 ff.
 and physics, 157
Purpose, the concept of, 38

Qualia, 26
Qualities
 of contents, 203
 division of, 6, 30
 evolution of, 207 f.
 and relations, 20 ff.
 of value, 90
Quality, 124, 182 ff.
 and interest, 99
 over-all, 228
 primary, 18, 97, 147, 200

secondary, 17, 19, 97, 200
simple, 142
tertiary, 97-98

Realism, 102
Realists, 91, 100
Red, 8, 10, 148, 172, 216-21, 253, 255
Redness, 45, 165, 249, 251
Reich, 281
Reiser, 281
Relations, internal and external, 12, 20 ff.
    and qualities, 26 ff., 28 n., 145 n.
Relativism, objective, 18 n.
Relativity of sense classifications, 74
    of aesthetic reactions, 184-85
Religion and the supersensible, 3, 271-72
Respects of color resemblance, 41, 43, 142
Response, 147
Rich, 274 n.
Richards, I. A., 28 n., 121 n., 162 n.
Rickert, 90
Ross, 164

Sampson, 15
Santayana, 21, 22, 175, 201
Scarlet, 218
Scheerer, 156 n.
Schopenhauer, 177 n., 212
Self, the, 101, 109, 112, 195-97
*Sensa*, 203-4
Sensation, 1-29, 115, 203, 252-53
    and affection, 57, 127, 130 ff.
    dimensional theories of, 146 ff.
    dimensions of, 209 ff., 224, 233-34, 238, 241
    and feeling, 13, 37, 107-17, 122, 128, 133, 135-37
    and knowing, 36-37
    thermal, 259 ff.
Sense qualities and adaptation, 250 ff.
Similarity and harmony, 166-67, 225-26
Skin sensations, 234
Smells, 258
Sociality, 13, 19-20, 33, 101-2, 112-14, 192 ff., 245
Soul, 109-10
Sound, 225 ff., 257

Sounds, 59 ff., 66, 189
    and colors, 62, 67, 75, 78, 79, 81, 84
Souriau, E., 182 n.
Space, 66, 196 ff., 264 n.
Spearman, 106, 136
Spencer, 144
Spiral of sounds, 226, 228 ff., 233
Spiritualism, 16, 101
Spranger, 107
Steger, 271 n.
Stein, L., 91 n.
Stern, 85
Stevens, 64 n.
*Stimmung*, of colors, 175
Stout, 24 n., 140-42
Strong, 50, 76, 144
Stumpf, 65 n.
Sweetness, 201-2, 204, 250
Sympathy, 13, 246
Synesthesia, 77-85

Taste and smell, 236 ff., 261
Taylor, C. D., 60 n.
Techoueyres, 25
Temperature, 75
Tertiary quality, 97
Theology, 271
Three-process theory of vision, the, 223 n.
Thurstone, 107, 112-13
Timbre, 228, 233
Titchener, 61, 115, 135, 201
Tonality, 125
Tone color, 65, 231
Tones, 59, 166, 228, 232, 233, 267
Tornay, 240 n.
Transmutation, 248 n.
Troland, 67 n., 73 n., 138, 152, 215, 224, 228, 232, 251 n., 260, 265 n., 274

Vagueness, 175, 207 f.
    as criterion of feeling, 131
Valentine, 117 n.
Value, 89, 98-99, 102, 187
Variables
    in sensation, 241
    of sound, 65

Variation, 190
Violet, 215, 218, 221, 225
Vision, 64, 223 n.
   and behavior, 253
Visual timbre, 227
Volkelt, 182 n.
Volley effect, 70
Volume in sounds, 66, 67 n.
Vowel quality, 229

Warmth, 204, 216, 233, 267
Wave-packet, 25, 145
Weiss, 267 n.

Wellek, 85 n.
Werner, H., 85 n., 104 n.
Wever-Bray experiment, the, 67 n., 70, 72
Wheeler, 65 n., 82–83
White, 170, 209, 225, 253
Whitehead, 7, 36 n., 94 n., 101 n., 155 n., 181, 248 n., 281
Wood, 28, 162
Wundt, 8

Yellow, 7, 119, 148, 184, 216–21, 253
Youtz, 188 n.

Zietz, 83–85

www.ingramcontent.com/pod-product-compliance
Lightning Source LLC
Chambersburg PA
CBHW070235230426
43664CB00014B/2305